What in the World are COVID vaccines

What in the World are COVID vaccines

Dr. Austin Mardon, Kelsey Goddard, Bhargavi Venkataraman, Ananna Arna, Ida Marchese, Terrence Wu, Cynthia Xu, Suhel Sadik Patel, Yash Joshi, Marcey Costello, Armita Yousefi, Dasarathy Mutharasan

2021

GM
PRESS

Typeset and Cover Design by Brett Boyd

ISBN: 978-1-77369-243-2
Golden Meteorite Press
103 11919 82 St NW
Edmonton, AB T5B 2W3
www.goldenmeteoritepress.com

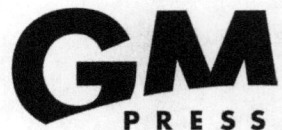

GM
PRESS

Introduction

Ivy Truong

A LITTLE MORE THAN a year into the COVID-19 pandemic, there have been 153 million confirmed cases and 3.2 million deaths. The disease caused by the SARS-Coronavirus 2 is incredibly infectious, with the median R0 value being 5.7 — any person with COVID-19 can potentially transmit the coronavirus to 5 or 6 people (*Ramirez & Biggers, 2020*). As the coronavirus began to rapidly spread from Wuhan, Hubei onto the global scene, the race between the virus and the medical community commenced. Research efforts for a COVID-19 vaccine roll across Novavax, AstraZeneca, Johnson & Jonhson, and other pharmaceutical giants present vaccine candidates, each a little different from the other.

The rush to produce an effective vaccine against the rapidly spreading virus plays a key role in the synthesis of a new type of vaccine — mRNA vaccines. With the pressing time constraint, the emergence of mRNA vaccines is incredibly important due to its swift development time. Conventional vaccines attenuated forms of the pathogen injected into the host to trigger an immune response, producing memory cells in the event of exposure to the actual form of the virus. This requires complex processes of growing and harvesting the pathogen in the lab, with some more difficult processes requiring the regeneration of a recombinant protein derived from the virus (*College of Physicians of Philadelphia, 2000*), which poses a biohazard risk and consumes a large amount of time. In the case of SARS-CoV2, the conventional vaccine development strategies are no longer effective in keeping pace with its infectious ability and speed. Combating COVID-19 outbreaks would require a novel method of vaccine production that does not require the numerous steps that would delay vaccine development. The vaccines highlighted in this book are the Pfizer-BioNTech, Moderna, AstraZeneca, and Sputnik vaccines. This range of vaccines differ in various aspects, most notably, they are different types of vaccines. The Pfizer and Moderna vaccines are revolutionary in that they are mRNA vaccines, the new type of vaccine that confers immunity in a completely different way from traditional vaccines. The most current mRNA vaccines, BNT162b2 (Pfizer)and mRNA-1273 (Moderna) both target the same virus, which can provide an enormous amount of insight on the mRNA vaccination development and the resulting efficacy of mRNA vaccines. Comparison of the two mRNA vaccines allows us to determine the best design features for an mRNA vaccine. Both mRNA vaccines target the same SARS-CoV2 antigen and produce the mRNA molecule that codes for the antigen transmembrane spike protein (S-protein) that on the virus, allows for the penetration and infection of host cells (*Corbett et al., 2020*). The S-protein is then synthesized in the host body to trigger the immune response, and produce antibodies against the actual virus (*Verbeke et al., 2021*). While both mRNA and conventional vaccines make use of the host's innate immunity, the mRNA vaccination bypasses the arduous processes of harvesting and processing attenuated pathogens. Comparing this new class of vaccine products to conventional vaccines such as AstraZeneca and Sputnik's, which all focus on the same disease target presents further knowledge on effectual vaccines and emphasizes the changes in vaccine development in the emergence of new pathogens.

Even with the increasing speed of vaccine development and approval by the U.S. Food and Drug Administration and Health Canada, the main problem lies within the distribution of the vaccines. The delay in allocating vaccines to most regions of the globe plays a devastating effect on the continued spread of SARS-CoV2. Vaccinations impede the virus' transmission, utilizing herd immunity to defer and eventually block off the spread of the virus. As the coronavirus is easily spread throughout the population and more people are infected, the likelihood of significant mutations is drastically increased. A key example of this is the D614G mutation in the SARS-CoV2 spike protein that increases infectivity by reducing the shedding of the spike protein that prevents the virus from penetrating the host cell (*Zhang et al., 2020*). All the mRNA vaccines code for the spike protein, thus, changes in the spike protein could render the body's antibodies ineffective against the new SARS-CoV2 variants. The spike protein would have changed to such an extent that is no longer recognizable by the immune system, thus rendering the vaccine ineffectual. Several COVID-19 variants that are of concern; B.1.1.7 variant, B.1.351 variant, P.1 variant, B.1.427, and B.1.429 variants all spread at a higher rate and with more ease than any other variants (*CDC, 2020*), thus posing a risk for increased transmission speed and imposing a more pressing time constraint for vaccine development and distribution. As of the time of publication, the current vaccines are generally effective against these variants, but due to the increased transmission and thus increased probability of mutation, it is only time before the antibodies generated by the vaccines no longer recognize the COVID-19 variants.

The purpose of introducing vaccines to a population is to achieve herd immunity, ideally, a large enough proportion of the population should be immune to the target virus to offer enough protection that impedes transmission. For the coronavirus, 67% to 80% of the population must be vaccinated to reduce the spread of the disease to a controllable state (*Randolph & Barreiro, 2020*). Understanding the population's attitude towards vaccines is crucial in developing a vaccination programme. A major focus of an effective vaccination programme would be the representation of vaccines, the advancements in communicative platforms can be an influential method of presenting information campaigns targeting the varying reasons for vaccine hesitancy across different demographics. While a major player in vaccine hesitancy is misinformation and the lack of credible and correct information, the behaviours that drive the concern for vaccinations have underlying reasons that differ across different groups of people. It is important to understand the reasons why or how certain misinformation materializes and circulates in certain groups to change how vaccines are represented, targeting the different root causes of vaccine hesitancy among individual groups. While the development of effective vaccines is important, the allocation process plays a large factor in confronting the outbreak. Vaccine hesitancy stems from a complex background and is often contextually specific. For example, in the H1N1 pandemic of 2009, there was a perception that the vaccine was unsafe due to its rushed development, similar to the major concerns surrounding the COVID-19 vaccines (*Mills et al., 2020*).

Throughout history, in the face of extreme anxiety, conspiracy theories materialize to maintain a sense of control and stability for some groups of people (*Douglas et al., 2017*). This behaviour is mirrored in the COVID-19 outbreak where financial, social, and political stress is particularly detrimental to the psychological state of the population, varying depending on the intensity and types of groups affected by the stress. It is important to define the difference between conspiracy theories and vaccine hesitancy, vaccine hesitancy stems from a place of understandable concerns and misinformation such as potential conflicts of interest, development time, new scientific developments, etc. Conspiracy theories are a set of false beliefs surrounding a situation supported by a plethora of incorrect information supporting the belief. Anti-vaccine beliefs have existed far before the outbreak, previously circulating in just niche communities, but in the wake of an outbreak where the topic of vaccines has surfaced, discussion promoting harmful beliefs based on theoretical beliefs have increased outside the niche groups. Outlandish theories such as the 'microchip conspiracy' and 'Pandemic' that were once absurd are increasing in engagement (*Ullah et al., 2021*), notably on online platforms. The major concern with conspiracies, especially the increase during a pandemic is the potential of mass vaccine refusal, leading to a prolonged outbreak and risk of more potent mutants emerging. It is important to address the root of these conspiracies and the false beliefs that they are built on. Furthermore, focusing on the causes of anxiety in particularly targeted groups is critical in reversing the attitudes and false beliefs of vaccines.

Prolonging a 'syndemic' epidemic such as COVID-19 only further exacerbates the detrimental effects of the disease, not only by direct illness but also by amplifying the non-communicable diseases and worsening social conditions. Rapid vaccine development is a necessity, and the synthesis of new mRNA vaccines for the same disease target that skips some of the processes in conventional vaccines gives rise to the possibility of eliminating the virus sooner than expected. The mRNA vaccines Pfizer and Moderna can be compared to conventional vaccines AstraZeneca and Sputnik, which all focus on the same disease target, providing insight on the efficacy of the new vaccine technology. Although the development of a new vaccine strategy is revolutionary, vaccine hesitancy arises from the lack of knowledge regarding the technological advancements, contributing to the prolonging of vaccinations and thus the pandemic. Along the road, conspiracy theories based on incorrect beliefs also impede the development of herd immunity among the population, confronting the complex root causes of vaccine refusal due to vaccine hesitancy and conspiracy theories is crucial in ensuring the circulation of vaccines and stopping the transmission of coronavirus.

Ivy Truong

Chapter 1

HISTORY OF VIRAL VACCINATION

Kelsey Goddard

Origins of inoculation

EARLY MEDICINE AND vaccination reflected many societies' balancing of the magical, the superstitious, and the scientific in healing their ill and preventing societal devastation at the hands of epidemics. While vaccinations today target a whole host of different diseases and their variants, for centuries the focus of the quest for immunity was smallpox.

This highly infectious disease caused a fever and disfiguring skin rash, and appears as far back as Egypt in 1570 to 1085 BC (*Riedel, 2005*). The smallpox plague of Antonine in the Roman Empire killed almost 7 million people, with 2,000 people dying per day when the disease was at its most virulent (*Riedel, 2005; Watts, 2020*). 18th century England reported 400,000 people dying annually of smallpox, with a third of its survivors blinded and even more with pitted scars. It travelled many continents thanks to war, exploration, and trade, resulting in, for instance, the infection of the Aztecs and the Incas by the Spanish and Portuguese conquistadors. Needless to say, the danger of the disease was well understood by the populations it tore through, and so it was even used as a weapon by the British to devastate

Indigenous populations (*Riedel, 2005*).

It would take until 1980 for the World Health Organisation [WHO] to call smallpox eradicated, a distinction that belongs to no other disease. The vaccine's origin is often accredited to Gloucestershire native Edward Jenner in 1796, but the prevalence of smallpox meant vaccinations were taking place long before his invention (*Riedel, 2005*).

Superstition often tangled with science. A doctor in the 1600s tended to victims of smallpox "by allowing no fire in the room, leaving the windows permanently open, drawing the bedclothes no higher than the patient's waist, and administering 'twelve bottles of small beer every twenty-four hours'" (*Riedel, 2005*). However, there was a rudimentary understanding of immunity: as far back as 430 BC, smallpox survivors tended to its victims. Inoculation was a process wherein the disease's physical symptoms, such as the scabs, were touched or ingested to build up immunity. It was used in Africa, India, China, parts of the Ottoman Empire, and Europe long before Jenner made his own attempt (*Boylston, 2012; Riedel, 2005*). In some parts of Europe, Africa, and Asia was a practice called "buying the pocks," wherein people would pay to touch scabs and smallpox-infected clothing or wool (*Boylston, 2012*).

A letter from Cassem Algaida Aga, the ambassador from Tripoli, Libya, to the Court of St. James during the 1700s, wrote: "*this practice is so innocent, and so sure, that out of a hundred persons inoculated not two die; whereas on the contrary, out of a hundred persons that are infected with the small-pox the natural way, there die commonly about thirty*" (*Boylston, 2012*).

In April 1721, Lady Mary Wortley Montague, wife of a British diplomat, had her two children treated in this fashion. The doctor, Charles Maitland, was subsequently granted the royal license to inoculate prisoners and orphaned children. The subjects were made entirely immune to smallpox, but society truly gained new appreciation for the practice when Maitland inoculated the daughters of the Princess of Wales. Once inoculation became commonplace, it was not without its complications (2% to 3% of patients died from the disease, infected others, or suffered from other diseases that were transferred in the process), but its promise of long-awaited relief to society would catch the attention of Edward Jenner (*Boylston, 2012; Riedel, 2005*).

The inoculation procedure previously described used scabs or fluids from smallpox-infected humans. However, Jenner had heard of dairymaids who, once infected with their cows' smallpox variant, were made immune to smallpox in general. This "cowpox" was a fairly mild illness whose udder sores transferred to humans, as was the case with dairymaid Sarah Nelms. In 1796, Jenner used Nelms' sores to inoculate a boy named James Phipps. He had mild symptoms for nine days, but on the tenth he recovered and remained healthy after exposure to smallpox. He named the successful process vaccination, after the Latin word for cow, vacca, and cowpox, vaccinia (*The College of Physicians of Philadelphia [CPP], n.d.; Riedel, 2005*).

Even as vaccines became safer and more effective, smallpox would occasionally return (*Britannica, n.d.*). When it was rediscovered in New York City in 1947, health commissioners and the government worked together to vaccinate 80% of the city. The epidemic came to a sudden halt because of the successful campaign: it infected only twelve people and killed two (*CPP, n.d.*). In 1967, the Intensified Smallpox Eradication Programme was launched by the WHO in Africa, Asia, and Brazil. Despite the WHO allegedly using coercion to ensure vaccination, in 1980 the disease was declared eradicated. In 1990, the United States military ceased vaccinating soldiers for smallpox – a notable milestone, considering the long battle between militaries and infectious diseases (*CPP, n.d.*).

Wartime developments

After Jenner, the science of vaccination made vast and promising developments. The availability of the electron microscope and the ability to safely grow viruses in laboratories introduced the first steps of whole inactivated vaccines. These involve a virus made unable to infect through chemical or physical methods, such as formaldehyde, heat, or gamma irradiation (*Britannica, n.d.; Sanders et al., 2014*). In 1886, Daniel Elmer Salmon and Theobald Smith immunized pigeons of cholera with a whole inactivated vaccine derived from hog cholera. Eventually, inactivated vaccines were created for typhoid fever, rabies, and cholera (*Sanders et al., 2014*). Vaccine development for aggressive diseases of the time, such as the aforementioned typhoid, would be prompted by World War I and II's skyrocketing infection rate (*Hoyt, 2006*).

Tetanus, influenza, and typhoid fever vaccines were all in progress more than 30 years before World War I. The close quarters of military camps, travel to unfamiliar locations, unhygienic combat locations, and open wounds were all responsible for the prevalence of these diseases during the wars (*Wever & van Bergen, 2012*). Citizens were also at risk. In World War II, Europe saw 1 million cases of diphtheria and 50,000 deaths, and in World War I, it is estimated that influenza, not direct combat, caused nearly 80% of casualties in the United States Army (*CPP, n.d.; Hoyt, 2006*).

Typhoid fever was prevalent in the Second Boer War, the Spanish-American War, and South African War during the late 1800s (*Britannica, n.d.; CPP, n.d.*). Out of 57,684 cases of typhoid in the South African War's British troops, 9,022 soldiers died. Almroth Wright's typhoid vaccine was trialed in the Indian army and then introduced to the British, but only 14,626 men out of 328,244 volunteered for the vaccine. Consequently, the benefits of Wright's vaccine would only reveal themselves with World War I: while the infection rate during the South African War was 105 per 1,000 troops, in World War I it was 2.35 out of 1,000. The death rate plummeted from 14.6 per 1,000, to 0.139 (*Britannica, n.d.*). In World War II, the U.S. Army Medical Department said that among their troops, typhoid had nearly entirely disappeared (*CPP, n.d.*).

Emil von Behring and Shibasaburo Kitasato created a vaccine for tetanus between 1890 and 1892 which was given to wounded soldiers during World War I (*Britannica, n.d.; Wever & van Bergen, 2012*). As a result, tetanus's tenacity dwindled, but this vaccine was not without risks. Anaphylaxis in response to the vaccine killed many, despite the uncountable soldiers the vaccine saved from tetanus. Public doubt followed these lethal side effects, but a combination of the vaccine and improved knowledge and technologies in surgeries, cleaning, and wound-draining resulted in a steep decline in tetanus by 1914 (*Wever & van Bergen, 2012*). A more efficient and safe vaccine was rolled out for World War II (*Britannica, n.d.*).

Other vaccines that were greatly improved throughout World War II were those for yellow fever, cholera and smallpox. Wartime programs and funding saw the creation of a new typhus vaccine, botulinum toxoid, and Japanese encephalitis vaccine. Vaccines for influenza, pneumococcal pneumonia, and the plague were licensed for the first time. The first double-blind randomized clinical trial for a pneumococcal vaccine enrolled over 17,000 men from the Army Air Force Technical School. The vaccination trials for influenza in the military provided vital data, and within two years, the combined effort, participation and funding resulted in the first effective vaccine against influenza being administered for the general public (*Hoyt, 2006*).

Besides increases in funding (funding for US Army medical

research increased by over 100 percent during World War II), the USA Army Epidemiology Board was founded to oversee commissions on various diseases such as air-borne infections, neurotropic virus diseases, and pneumonia. 10 commissions of 100 civilian scientists were enlisted through the Preventative Medicine Division to "conduct research on diseases of military importance" (*Hoyt, 2006*).

Polio

Polio was a great concern in North America in the early-to-mid 1900s. The disease mainly targeted children under five, but regardless of age, it often caused life-long physical disabilities, paralysis, or death. In the United States during 1952 alone, there were 57,628 cases with 21,000 resulting in paralysis. Between 1949 and 1954, approximately 11,000 Canadians were paralyzed by polio and hundreds more died (*Canadian Public Health Association, n.d.; CPP, n.d.*).

In 1935, John Kolmer tested a live attenuated vaccine on about 10,000 children (*CPP, n.d.*). While inactivated vaccines use a neutralized virus, live attenuated vaccines contain live viruses that are weakened in a laboratory. The immune system learns how to eliminate this weakened virus, but since the virus is still active, they are considered a higher risk vaccine (*Li et al., 2020*). Kolmer's tests resulted in several subjects dying of polio, paralyzed, or otherwise made ill (*CPP, n.d.*).

Despite this, live attenuated vaccines for polio continued to be developed because of their benefits: if all risks are mitigated, the immune system will almost certainly learn how to fight off the virus (*Li et al., 2020*). In 1948, Hilary Koprowski drank his live attenuated vaccine to prove its safety before testing it on 20 children in a facility for intellectually disabled children and children with epilepsy. They all remained healthy and developed antibodies to fight polio (*CPP, n.d.*).

Jonas Salk and Albert Bruce Sabin created two different polio vaccines that reached the public in the 1950's and 1960's, and are known today for both their contributions and a devastating incident that damaged public trust in polio vaccines. In 1952, Salk tested his inactivated vaccine on physically and intellectually disabled children. Perhaps to mitigate doubt lingering from previous vaccination disasters, Salk injected himself and his family with the vaccine (*CPP, n.d.*). In 1954, the Vaccine Advisory Committee delivered Salk's vaccine to a remarkable 1.3 million participants in a field trial. About 650,000 children were vaccinated or given a placebo, while the remaining children were untreated and observed for general polio infection (*CPP, n.d.; Kurlander & Juhl, 2020*). A year of studies confirmed that the vaccine was 80-90% effective, so it was swiftly licensed by the U.S. government (*CPP, n.d.*).

Only weeks later, vaccinated children were infected with polio. All paralysis symptoms originated in the vaccinated arm while polio usually began its process in the legs. The mass vaccination rollouts were abruptly cancelled. The vaccines given to the ill were traced back to Cutter Laboratories and the resulting 40 000 cases of polio, 200 cases of paralysis, and ten deaths defined what is now called the Cutter incident. However, the failure was likely due to the inexperience of that particular laboratory and not the inefficacy of Salk's vaccine itself (*CPP, n.d.; Fitzpatrick, 2006*).

After installing rigorous new vaccine regulations which remain today, public vaccination resumed, but some locations refused to participate. The Polio Vaccination Assistance Act of 1955 reserved $30 million to distribute Salk's polio vaccines to an eventual 30 million American children (*CPP, n.d.; Kurlander & Juhl, 2020*).

Sabin was busy improving his live attenuated polio vaccine, and by 1959, it was given to 10 million children in the USSR. By the early 1960s, his licensed vaccines would protect against all three types of poliovirus. However, Sabin's vaccines were also not without mistrust: they also resulted in sporadic cases of paralysis and polio throughout the 1980's and 1990's. The advantages and disadvantages of Sabin and Salk's vaccines continue to be discussed (*CPP, n.d.; Fitzpatrick, 2006*).

The challenges and tragedies were ultimately not in vain: by 1994, both North and South America were declared free of polio (*CPP, n.d.*). In part because of the lawsuits from the Cutter incident, in 1986 the National Vaccine Injury Compensation Program was created to "protect vaccine manufacturers from litigation on a scale that [threatens] the continuing production of vaccines" (*Fitzpatrick, 2006*). Around the world, efforts to eliminate polio continued, with the late 90s seeing the vaccination of around 250 million children in India and expanded vaccination efforts in Sudan. Eventually, at the turn of the century, polio cases had plummeted 99% worldwide (*CPP, n.d.*).

SARS-CoV-1 and MERS-CoV

COVID-19 is not the first time a coronavirus was brought to global attention. Beginning in the Guangdong province of China in 2002, SARS-CoV-1 spread through five continents and 33 countries, resulting in 8,450 cases and 810 deaths (*Jiang et al., 2005*). The United States only saw about 29 cases, and in mid-2003 the concern over the virus was brought to a swift end when the World Health Organisation announced that the epidemic, small as it seems now, was over (*Roossinck, 2020*). While variations on the virus would appear again in Guangdong in early 2004, SARS-CoV-1 would not spread with the speed it did between 2002 and 2003. Consequently, all in-progress vaccines were never licensed (*Roossinck, 2020*). Despite that, Jiang et al.'s 2005 article speaks to SARS-CoV-1 in a way that now rings prophetic: "*a SARS epidemic may recur at any time in the future, either by the virus escaping from laboratory samples or by SARS-CoV isolates evolving from SARS-CoV-like virus in animal hosts.*"

SARS-CoV-1 (Severe Acute Respiratory Syndrome Coronavirus) was followed in 2012 by its cousin, MERS-CoV (Middle East Respiratory Syndrome Coronavirus). MERS-CoV caused outbreaks in Saudi Arabia in 2012 and 2015, as well as in South Korea in 2015. Unlike SARS-CoV-1, it occasionally resurfaces: in January 2020 there were 2,519 cases across 27 countries with a 35% mortality rate (*Li et al., 2020*).

Testing for a vaccine began soon after both outbreaks. Various methods were attempted for SARS-CoV-1, including virus-like particle vaccines, DNA vaccines, viral vector vaccines, whole inactivated vaccines, and live attenuated vaccines, but it was the protein subunit vaccines that proved most effective for SARS-CoV-1. The virus uses its S glycoprotein to invade host cells, and so these vaccines targeted that glycoprotein. Protein subunit vaccines were only joined in clinical stages by DNA vaccines and whole inactivated vaccines, but reports vary as to how much testing was done. Ultimately, it is certain that none were licensed or FDA approved, and no tests were done on humans (*Li et al., 2020; Padron-Regalado, 2020; Roossinck, 2020*). In the case of MERS-CoV, the DNA-based vaccine has been tested in clinical trials, while others are still being tested as of April 2020 (*Padron-Regalado, 2020*).

Reports vary on why SARS-CoV-1 or MERS-CoV-1 vaccines were not licensed, as well as on the effectiveness of the many vaccines made for these two diseases. In the case of SARS-CoV-1, it's very likely that the reason was as simple as it was no longer needed: the disease vanished after rigorous quarantining of the infected, aided by the disease's quick display of symptoms and lack of asymptomatic carriers unlike COVID-19 (*Roossinck, 2020*). Additionally, there was a high risk in exposing even vaccinated individuals to the virus, so the efficacy of the vaccines remains a mystery (*Padron-Regalado, 2020*). The vaccines created were over-all effective in animals, but did occasionally result in immune diseases and serious complications in the lungs. Meanwhile, MERS-CoV vaccine developments were likely delayed because of the difficulty in acquiring animals to test on (*Li et al., 2020; Padron-Regalado, 2020; Roossinck, 2020*).

Valuable information from these tests remain, however. While it is generally less effective than other protein-based vaccines, an N protein-based vaccine showed potential for a universal coronavirus vaccine. It was discovered that the E protein was most responsible for the inflammation of the lungs, and so it is predicted that in live attenuated vaccines, removing the E protein will greatly reduce the severity of infection. In fact, SARS-CoV-1 mutations completely missing the E proteins could protect hamsters against SARS-CoV-1 itself. RBD-based (recep-tor-binding domain based) vaccines greatly protected mice and even induced S-specific antibodies, which can potentially be replicated for variations on SARS-CoV-1. Also valuable are the reports on what proteins in SARS-CoV-1 and MERS-CoV did not result in protective immunity or neutralizing antibodies (*Li et al, 2020; Padron-Regalado, 2020*).

SARS-CoV-1 vaccines may have never made it to the public, and in most cases never made it to trial, but various COVID-19 vaccines are developing with unprecedented speed thanks to the centuries of aforementioned research behind them. Nucleic acid vaccines and viral vector vaccines were in use during recent influenza, Ebola, and Zika outbreaks, and so are taking a strong role in COVID-19 vaccine development. To save time, some

COVID-19 vaccines are sent to clinical trials without complete data from their animal trials, with trials being held in parallel fashion rather than one step at a time (*Li et al., 2020*). The severity of COVID-19's virulence as well as centuries of vaccine research and innovation promises a landscape of varied, complex, and urgent vaccine development on a global scale.

mRNA

mRNA vaccines are one of the newest types of vaccines to protect against serious developing diseases. They differ from most of the previously discussed vaccines in that they don't involve an altered or weakened version of the virus itself, and as a result present no risk of infecting the patient (*Centers for Disease Control and Prevention, 2021; Pardi et al., 2018*). More on this vaccine and its use for COVID-19 will be discussed in a later chapter.

mRNA's ability to teach cells to create certain proteins was first tested in the early 1970s. In the next couple decades it was considered potentially useful for protein replacement therapies, though the adaptations to mRNA that would most benefit its therapeutic abilities could possibly hinder its potential as a vaccine. Overall, mRNA had great potential and represented reassuring progress in the field of vaccines, but was extremely sensitive when being engineered and maintained (*Pardi et al., 2018; Schlake et al., 2012; Zhang et al., 2019*).

In 1990, mice injected with reporter gene mRNAs proved that it was possible to use in vitro transcribed mRNA in animals; even more promising was that the mice muscle cells acquired the mRNA without requiring any special delivery systems in the serum. A couple years later, it was proved that these effects could elicit responses in the hypothalamus of rats. Despite the industry continuing to focus on DNA-based and protein-based vaccines, mRNA would soon be advocated as a strong contender for vaccine creation because of its adaptability, ability to be easily and affordably reproduced at short notice, and safety for patients because of its lack of infecting agents (*Pardi et al., 2018; Schlake et al., 2012*).

In the 2000s, mRNA vaccines appeared more frequently in various vaccine trials. mRNAs are very sensitive to temperature changes, and so developments have been made to mitigate that risk (*Schlake et al., 2012; Zhang et al., 2019*). They would go on to be a part of the effort, whether licensed or in clinical trials, for influenza, Zika, and rabies, as well as cancer clinical trials (*Centers for Disease Control and Prevention, 2021; Schlake et al., 2012*).

Unanswered questions & future directions

Vaccines for dozens of other infectious and deadly diseases were developed, tested, and licensed alongside and between the success stories previously described. From "buying the pocks" to mRNA vaccines, the safety, understanding, efficiency, and especially the speed of invention and production of vaccines have all increased to improve global health and peace of mind. Smallpox took thousands of years of lucky happenstance and ingenuity before a vaccine was licensed. In comparison, COVID-19 ravaged the globe for barely a year before vaccine options were rolled out: effective, rigorously monitored, and widely-available. Perhaps COVID-19 will one day reach complete eradication like smallpox, but that is only one of many questions on people's minds regarding COVID-19 vaccination.

History does not only reveal vaccine successes. As efficient and strict as vaccine standards are, unprecedented complications can arise even after multiple trials of testing and decades of research. The Cutter incident has been discussed, but it is joined by swine flu vaccinations in 1977 that caused increased risk of Guillain-Barré syndrome while the swine flu never hit the emergency levels the vaccines were preparing for (*CPP, n.d.*). 1963 saw a measles vaccine which made patients vulnerable to a measles mutation that was more severe than the type for which they were vaccinated (*Sanders et al., 2014*). The 1930 Lübeck disaster describes tuberculosis vaccines in Germany that were accidentally contaminated with unaltered and infectious tuberculosis. Although the vaccine itself was greatly effective and later promoted by the International Tuberculosis Campaign, the 73 deaths of 249 vaccinated infants incited controversy and fear (*Britannica, n.d.; CPP, n.d.*). This is nothing to say of potential distrust of the industry for their history of testing on children in sensitive circumstances where they cannot consent.

It is uncertain what the long-term effects of COVID-19's many varied vaccines will be, and how to balance those risks with the present, severe risks of COVID-19 itself. For all the answers that history and empirical evidence can provide, diseases are often unpredictable because of their complexity and the complexity of the societies they infect. It is still puzzling why COVID-19 spread so rapidly and with such force, while its cousin SARS-CoV-1 was eliminated before a vaccine was even created and MERS-CoV still infects people in 2020 yet has never reached pandemic levels.

There are incredible scientific successes throughout history when it comes to producing effective vaccines and eliminating diseases, even in part; however, there are also unpredictable tragedies and scientific complications. Where COVID-19 will fit in our world's history of vaccines is perhaps the biggest question of all.

Chapter 2

Overview of COVID-19

Bhargavi Venkataraman

Origin

CORONAVIRUS DISEASE (COVID-19), formerly known as 2019 novel coronavirus, is a severe acute respiratory syndrome that was first identified in Wuhan, Hubei Province, China in December 2019 (*CDC, 2020*). At this time, health authorities in China reported a pneumonia outbreak of unknown origin and of the first 27 documented hospitalized patients, the majority of the cases were connected to Huanan Seafood Wholesale Market (*Hu et al., 2020*). Through the use of RNA sequencing and isolation of the virus from the bronchoalveolar lavage fluid samples obtained from patients, Chinese scientists determined that the causative agent for the outbreak is a novel coronavirus (*Hu et al, 2020*). In the beginning of January 2020, China announced this etiological identification publicly and by the end of the month, the World Health Organization (WHO) declared a Public Health Emergency of International Concern (PHEIC) alert (*Hu et al., 2020*). In March 2020, the WHO officially identified COVID-19 as a pandemic and since this point, the virus has spread to all continents, causing thousands of deaths globally (*Hu et al., 2020*).

Structure

The virus has a spherical shape and is named "corona" for the crown-like spike proteins on its outer surface (*Shereen et al., 2020*). It is minute in size, being only 65 to 125 nanometers in diameter, and contains an enveloped, positive single-stranded RNA as nucleic matter (*Shereen et al., 2020*). Coronaviruses are part of the Coronaviridae family in the Nidovirales order and belong to the Orthocoronavirinae subfamily (*Li et al., 2020*). Within this subfamily, there are four genera: alphacoronavirus, betacoronavirus, gammacoronavirus and deltacoronavirus (*Li et al., 2020*). SARS-CoV-2 is a betacoronavirus, like the first severe acute respiratory syndrome (SARS) and the Middle East respiratory syndrome (MERS) which caused viral pneumonia outbreaks in China in 2002 and in Saudi Arabia in 2012 respectively (*Li et al., 2020*). SARS-CoV-2 shares 79% genome sequence identity with SARS-CoV and 50% genome sequence identity with MERS-CoV. SARS-CoV-2, SARS-CoV and MERS-CoV are all thought to have originated from bats and then infected humans through transmission from intermediary animal carriers (*Li et al., Tang, 2020*). Accordingly, the closest relative to SARS-CoV-2 is a bat coronavirus called RaTG13, first identified in Yunnan province, China (*Hu et al., 2020*). Its full genome sequence is 96.2% identical to SARS-CoV-2's genome sequence identity, making it have the greatest genetic similarity to SARS-CoV-2 (Hu et al., 2020).

Variants

Since the first report of the coronavirus in China, other variants of the virus have been reported around the world (*"New Variants of Coronavirus: What You Should Know", n.d.*). Variants of the virus occur when the virus' genes become mutated, as is common with RNA viruses like the coronavirus, and are often a result of geographic separation (*"New Variants of Coronavirus: What You Should Know", n.d.*). One such mutated coronavirus variation is the B.1.1.7 variant in southeastern England, commonly referred to as the "UK strain", which has preliminary evidence showing that it is more contagious than previous coronaviruses (*Moore and Offit, 2021*). There is also another variant first identified in Brazil called P1 and a variant that first began circulating in southern California called CAL.20C (*Moore and Offit, 2021*). However, the most concerning variant is the N501Y.V2 variant first reported in South Africa which may be able to re-infect those who have already recovered from other versions of the coronavirus and thus, may be resistant to existing vaccines (*"New Variants of Coronavirus: What You Should Know", n.d.*). These variants have now been detected in numerous other countries around the world, including Canada. In Canada, they are considered "Variants of Concern" due to the genetic differences between the viruses posing significant clinical and public health concerns that affect transmissibility of the disease, virulence in individuals, effectiveness of previously tested vaccines and diagnostic testing standards (*COVID-19 Variants of Concern (VOCs), n.d.*).

Transmission

The SARS-CoV-2 virus has numerous modes of transmission including, but not limited to, respiratory droplets, close-contact, airborne, fecal-oral, conjunctival, fomite, bloodborne, sexual and zoonotic (*COVID-19 Routes of Transmission – What We Know So Far", n.d.*). It is suggested that infected individuals are most contagious approximately 2 days prior to when they start developing and exhibiting symptoms, in the early stages of their illness (*"Coronavirus disease (COVID-19): How is it transmitted?", n.d.*). Research is still being conducted to comprehend how those who do not develop any symptoms of the illness can still transmit the virus to others (*"Coronavirus disease (COVID-19): How is it transmitted?", n.d.*). Respiratory droplet transmission occurs primarily when liquid particles from the mouth or nose of an infected individual spread to others through the acts of coughing, sneezing, speaking, singing and breathing (*"Coronavirus disease (COVID-19): How is it transmitted?", n.d.*). The virus has a higher likelihood of spreading in this fashion when individuals are in close-contact, approximately in a 1-2 metre range, with each other (*"Coronavirus disease (COVID-19): How is it transmitted?", n.d.*). SARS-CoV-2 can also spread through airborne transmission and is considered an opportunistic infectious pathogen which indicates that non-airborne transmission is the norm but small respiratory droplet (aerosol) transmission can also occasionally occur if the circumstances are favourable (*COVID-19 Routes of Transmission – What We Know So Far", n.d.*). One such circumstance is in poor ventilation conditions where recirculation of unfiltered air could result in sufficient accumulation of aerosols that uninfected individuals could inhale (*COVID-19 Routes of Transmission – What We Know So Far", n.d.*). SARS-CoV-2 has also been uncovered in patients' stool and respiratory samples, suggesting that it can be transmitted through a fecal-oral route, but knowledge on this transmission route is limited (*Ciotti et al., 2019*). The conjunctiva, a tissue lining the interior of eyelids, is also known to have contained SARS-CoV-2 RNA in certain patients, indicating that this could be a possible site of initial infection (*COVID-19 Routes of Transmission – What We Know So Far", n.d.*). Although the possibility of this kind of transmission is extremely low, one study has even shown that tears and ocular secretions could carry the virus (*COVID-19 Routes of Transmission – What We Know So Far", n.d.*). Fomite transmission of COVID-19 is mostly understood through testing in laboratory-controlled settings and is considered a lower risk when compared to transmission via respiratory droplets or direct contact (*CDC, 2020*). SARS-CoV-2 is able to survive on various surfaces and objects like door handles, phones, glass surfaces, paper money, etc. but there has not yet been evidence of food-borne transmission (*COVID-19 Routes of Transmission – What We Know So Far", n.d.*). Transmission through blood, blood products and organs is also a possibility, although of extremely low probability (*COVID-19*

Routes of Transmission – What We Know So Far", n.d.). SARS-CoV-2 RNA has previously been detected in patients' blood, plasma and serum but bloodborne transmission mostly remains a theoretical possibility as scientists review various case reports (*COVID-19 Routes of Transmission – What We Know So Far", n.d.*). Sexual transmission through semen, vaginal secretions and urine during sexual activities involving oral-anal contact is a combination of direct contact and transmission through respiratory droplets (*COVID-19 Routes of Transmission – What We Know So Far", n.d.*). Although viral RNA and live virus have been detected in saliva, indicating that intimate contact is a possible source of transmission, the risk of the disease spreading through this method is very low (*COVID-19 Routes of Transmission – What We Know So Far", n.d.*). Lastly, there is some evidence regarding zoonotic transmission where the virus gets transferred from companion, domestic and wild animals to humans but once again, the risk of this type transmission is relatively low (*COVID-19 Routes of Transmission – What We Know So Far", n.d.*).

High Risk

Certain populations have a higher likelihood of getting coronavirus disease as a result of various risk factors. One such factor is age with middle aged and older adults being at a higher risk of developing serious symptoms and those aged 85 and above being at the highest risk of having critical symptoms of COVID-19 (*Mayo Clinic Staff, n.d.*). In certain studies, it has been found that males had a slightly higher incidence rate of severe COVID-19 disease (*Hu & Wang, 2021*). Pre-existing lung problems such as chronic obstructive pulmonary disease, lung cancer, cystic and pulmonary fibrosis and asthma are also risk factors due to COVID-19 targeting the lungs (*Mayo Clinic Staff, n.d.*). Similarly, heart diseases like cardiomyopathy, pulmonary hypertension, congenital heart disease, general heart failure and coronary artery disease put individuals at a higher risk for exhibiting serious

COVID-19 symptoms (*Mayo Clinic Staff, n.d.*). For both lung and heart issues, it is recommended that individuals continue to take medications as prescribed to keep symptoms as controlled as possible and to limit severity due to complications like elevated blood pressure (*Mayo Clinic Staff, n.d.*). Diabetes and obesity have been known to decrease the efficiency of people's immune system and diabetes also generally increases risk of infections, so individuals with these conditions have a higher likelihood of contracting the virus (*Mayo Clinic Staff, n.d.*). Cancer and blood disorders such as sickle cell anemia and thalassemia increase the chance of individuals having severe COVID-19 symptoms (*Mayo Clinic Staff, n.d.*). Conditions and treatments that weaken the immune system like chronic kidney/liver disease, organ and bone marrow transplants, HIV, AIDS, cancer treatments, and prolonged use of prednisone or other such drugs can all increase the likelihood of developing coronavirus disease (*Mayo Clinic Staff, n.d.*). In general, individuals with comorbidities and conditions that result in a weakened immune system are more likely to develop serious illness caused by the coronavirus (*Hu, Wang, 2021*). Besides age, gender and health conditions, certain occupations also put people at a higher risk for contracting COVID-19. Essential workers such as healthcare workers, food service staff, public transit workers, delivery workers, etc. are at a greater risk of getting COVID-19 due to working outside and having less opportunity to adhere to social distancing guidelines and follow other protective measures (*Roberts et al., 2020*).

Protection

The most optimal method to preventing illness is to not be exposed to the virus through following various protective measures. Individuals are encouraged to avoid large gatherings or areas with many people unless absolutely necessary and staying home if sick in order to avoid spreading infection to others (*Mayo Clinic Staff, n.d.*). Social distancing of approximately 6 feet or 2 metres is recommended between individuals and people outside of their household (*Tosh, n.d.*). In public areas, especially where social distancing is not possible or is challenging to maintain, wearing a non-medical cloth face mask can help reduce the spread from individuals who are not exhibiting symptoms of COVID-19 (*Tosh, n.d.*). It is also important to wash hands often with soap and water for a minimum of 20 seconds and use hand sanitizers which contain at least 60% alcohol to help prevent spread of infections (*Tosh, n.d.*). Avoiding crowds and not frequenting indoor areas with poor ventilation can help prevent airborne transmission and spread of the virus through close contact (*Tosh, n.d.*). Further general practices such as covering one's mouth and nose when coughing or sneezing, not touching eyes, nose and mouth frequently and cleaning and disinfecting surfaces that people have direct contact with help limit fomite and respiratory droplet transmission (*Tosh, n.d.*). Those who work in healthcare settings require personal protective equipment (PPE) which includes eye protection like goggles, a face shield, and a respirator that covers the mouth and nose (*Maragakis, 2020*). These can prevent respiratory droplets containing the virus from reaching healthcare professionals' eyes and mucus membranes (*Maragakis, 2020*).

Symptoms

The most common clinical symptoms of COVID-19 are fever, dry cough, fatigue, dyspnea (shortness of breath or "air hunger") and sputum (saliva and mucus mixture coughed up from the respiratory tract) (*Alimohamadi et al., 2020*). Other less prevalent symptoms include chest tightness, diarrhea, hemoptysis (coughing up of blood), headaches, and myalgia (muscle pain) (*Alimohamadi et al., 2020*). Some patients also report loss of taste or smell, nasal congestion, conjunctivitis (red eyes), sore throat, skin rash, nausea, irritability, chills, reduced consciousness relating to seizures, anxiety, depression, sleep disorders and even development of rare neurological complications like strokes, brain inflammation, delirium and nerve damage (*"Coronavirus disease (COVID-19)", n.d.*). Signs of very critical COVID-19 disease are shortness of breath, loss of appetite, deliriousness, continuous pain and pressure in the chest, loss of speech and/or movement and high temperature (*"Coronavirus disease (COVID-19)", n.d.*). In cases of individuals experiencing these severe symptoms, they are encouraged to call a healthcare provider, hotline or a health facility to get immediate medical care (*"Coronavirus disease (COVID-19)", n.d.*). Symptoms can range from mild to very serious with some individuals not exhibiting any signs of the illness at all (*"Coronavirus: What is it and how can I protect myself?", n.d.*). Symptoms generally appear anywhere between two to fourteen days after exposure to the virus (*"Coronavirus: What is it and how can I protect myself?", n.d.*).

Vaccines

COVID-19 vaccines give instructions to the body's immune system to recognize and build a defence against the coronavirus (*Canada, 2020*). Vaccination has been proven to reduce the severity of an illness if an individual contracts the virus (*Canada, 2020*). Vaccines help prevent individuals from contracting the illness, becoming critically ill or passing away due to the illness (*"Get the facts about COVID-19 vaccines", n.d.*). They also prevent individuals from spreading the virus to other people and replicating, contributing to herd immunity in a community (*"Get the facts about COVID-19 vaccines", n.d.*). There are two main types of vaccines; mRNA vaccines and viral vector vaccines. The mRNA vaccines provide instructions to an individual's own cells on how to construct a coronavirus protein that eventually triggers an immune response against the virus (*Canada, 2020*). Viral vector vaccines use a virus whose harmful entities have been removed to make coronavirus proteins in the body without resulting in disease (*Canada, 2020*). These proteins then trigger an immune response to help the body fight against COVID-19, similar to mRNA vaccines (*Canada, 2020*). There are two main mRNA vaccines which are in distribution around the world. The first is Pfizer-BioNTech which is said to be 95% effective against the coronavirus, is for people aged 16 and above and requires two doses preferably given 21 days apart (*"Get the facts about COVID-19 vaccines", n.d.*). The second is the Moderna vaccine which is said to be 94% effective in preventing COVID-19 symptoms, is for people aged 18 or older and requires two doses preferably 28 days apart (*"Get the facts about COVID-19 vaccines", n.d.*). There are also two main viral vector vaccines which are in distribution around the world. The first is AstraZeneca which is said to be approximately 62% effective in preventing COVID-19 symptoms, is for individuals aged 18 and older and requires 2 doses preferably 4 to 12 weeks apart (*Canada, 2021*). The second is Johnson & Johnson's Janssen vaccine which is 66% effective in preventing COVID-19 symptoms, 85% effective in preventing severe COVID-19 disease, is for those aged 18 and older and requires only one injection (*"Get the facts about COVID-19 vaccines", n.d.*). There is some controversy about the use of this vaccine due to it having the potential to increase the risk of individuals getting a rare blood clotting disorder, but many countries such as the United States of America and Canada still distribute it due to its benefits outweighing its risks (*"Get the facts about COVID-19 vaccines", n.d.*).

Unanswered Questions and Future Directions

As the coronavirus is still relatively new, there are numerous questions that plague scientists and the world about it. One of the major questions about the virus is regarding its origin. Although it is known that the virus originated in Wuhan, China, there are still questions about where exactly it came from within Wuhan, when it started circulating there and when it began spreading outside of China (*Mallapaty, 2021*). Another source of confusion is about the quantity of people who have been infected with COVID-19 around the world as some people do not exhibit symptoms of the disease so they might not have reported that they had it (*Dunham, 2020*). Moreover, as new variants are being frequently reported around the world, there are questions about their dangerousness and whether present vaccines will still work on these variants (*COVID-19 Variants of Concern (VOCs), n.d.*). Scientists are also still unaware about why the severity of the illness varies among individuals, what qualifiers confirm that someone is not infectious anymore, if people can develop a protective immunity to the virus and whether there are complications after recovery from the disease (*Dunham, 2020*). However, the biggest question that everyone wants an answer to is when will this pandemic end and will the virus ever disappear completely? Scientists are still unsure if the vaccines against the virus will ever be 100% effective or if they will be like the flu vaccine and significantly lower the risk of getting infected but never completely eliminate it (*Dunham, 2020*). The future is likely going to show public health interventions being improved in order to contain the COVID-19 epidemic. Testing, contact tracing, isolating those infected and regulation of self-quarantining will be improved and made more efficient in order to reduce new cases (*Khanna et al., 2020*). There will also be a lot of resources put into antibody testing to identify individuals who are already immune to the virus and to learn more about whether those who have already recovered from COVID-19 will be reinfected (*Khanna et al., 2020*). Further, external factors like temperature, season, and humidity are known to impact COVID-19 so information will be collected from different parts of the world to truly understand the influence of these factors in the COVID-19 outbreak (*Khanna et al., 2020*). Research about vaccines and novel treatment options will continue to improve on the deficiencies of the current vaccines and reveal more about their risks and side effects (*Khanna et al., 2020*). There are also some general future trends that scientists predict might result from the practices people have developed from this pandemic. In the future, countries will more strictly enforce social distancing measures, limit large crowd interactions and mandate hand-washing and wearing masks when meeting with others in order to significantly reduce case counts without depending on vaccines (*Scudellari, 2020*). This would mean a complete change in the next couple years in the culture of how people interact with others (*Scudellari, 2020*). Although the future direction of the pandemic is unknown, there are still some projections circulating about the worst and best case scenario in the evolution of the virus. The worst case scenario is that if protective measures are not followed and vaccines do not provide long term immunity, infections will continue to rise rapidly (*Scudellari, 2020*). The virus would extensively circulate and become endemic, similar to malaria which is preventable and treatable but still kills hundreds of thousands of people yearly (*Scudellari, 2020*). Conversely, the best case scenario could be that SARS-CoV-2 immunity is permanent and after the virus has swept the world, it will disappear, even without the use of vaccines (*Scudellari, 2020*). However, to determine which scenario will occur, more data needs to be collected about the virus and how various communities respond to it around the world over time.

Chapter 3

Cellular and Biochemical Overview of SARS-CoV-2 and its variants

Ananna Bhadra Arna

THE NOVEL SEVERE acute respiratory syndrome coronavirus 2 (SARS-CoV-2) gives rise to the Coronavirus Disease-2019 (COVID-19) pandemic across the globe that has claimed many lives. It is very crucial to understand the biochemical aspect of the virus to construct proper vaccination with high efficiency and specificity. However, it is even more significant to ensure vaccines stay relevant to the ongoing mutations of SARS-CoV-2 to lessen further damage that could have been possibly prevented with proper research and implementation.

Random mutation is an important characteristic of natural selection and an important driver of evolution. These mutations are never directed to bring forth a beneficial characteristic to the organism. As shown by the Lederberg experiment, the outcome of mutation does not dictate its frequency in a population or its rate in a generation (*"Mutations are random", 2021*). Consequently, these mutations can be advantageous, neutral, or deleterious in nature to the organism. It is this outcome that causes evolutionary contingency. Only the advantageous mutations will be selected for as they improve the chances of survival and reproduction in the organism, while the deleterious mutations are selected against. Silent mutations are synonymous genetic changes that are not accompanied by a phenotypic change. They are believed to be neutral in nature as their resultant amino acid sequence remains unaffected. However, recently it has been discovered that synonymous mutations at a specific locus may serve as evolutionary beneficial to an organism's survival (*Caspermeyer, 2016*). Mutation rate is often dependent on the type of environment the organism is at; thus, this error rate is a reflection of their lifestyle. If well-adapted to its environment, the organism has a higher rate of deleterious mutations, while the beneficial mutation rates are higher if the organism is newly introduced to the environment. (*Duffy, 2018*)

RNA virus SARS-CoV-2 has a high mutation rate.

RNA viruses are infamous for their genetic instability. After entering its host, the RNA virus replicates its genetic material (RNA) by hijacking the host's replication machinery to further infect the cell. RNA synthesis lacks the proofreading activity that ensures high fidelity in DNA replication and ends up mismatching the repair systems (Steinhauer et al., 1992). An enhanced level of genetic heterogeneity is observed in RNA viruses where mutations at different loci bring forth the same or similar phenotypic deficit(s). Their high mutation rate is often associated with their virulence and rapid evolution which provide them with selective advantage over their other related viruses. Their threshold for tolerating heritable perturbations and maintaining phenotypical constancy differ across the viruses; this is often termed as "genetic robustness" (*Visser et al., 2003*). Many RNA viruses have optimized this threshold to their maximum mutation rate without any deleterious mutations. (*Barr & Fearns, 2016, Duffy, 2018*)

All Variants are not Strains.

During this pandemic, as these terms were more often used to address the variety in genetic makeup of SARS-related coronavirus, they were used interchangeably in many contexts. It is important that we get a good handle on the two terminologies to better make sense of the world around us and stay current. While both strain and variant derive from the parental strain, they have different meanings. RNA viruses have a high mutation rate. Mutations in the genetic material give rise to many variants of the virus. A RNA virus is genetically diverse as they conform to a group of related variants rather than following a single genotype (*Barr & Fearns, 2016*). Difference in the mutation number across the variants can exist anywhere from single to multiple. However, a variant is only a strain if these genetic changes have led to change(s) in the behavior or phenotype of the RNA virus. This way, the term "variant" can be used more closely as they exist in abundance in RNA viruses, while "strain" should be used more carefully. (*Madzokere & Herrero, n.d.*)

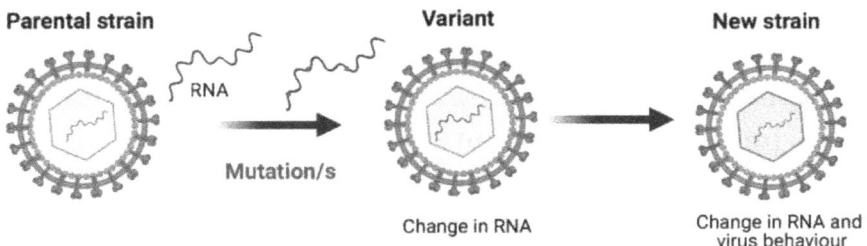

(*Viruses with mutations become variants. If the variant displays different physical properties to the original virus, we call it a new strain. Lara Herrero, created using BioRender, Author provided Madzokere & Herrero, n.d.*)

Homology between Severe acute respiratory syndrome-related coronavirus strains

SARS-CoV-2 is a member of the Coronaviridae family under the beta genus of the coronavirus sub-family. SARS-CoV-2 shares increasing homology with two other human-infecting coronaviruses of the genus: SARS-CoV and MERS-CoV. Coronaviruses have the largest genome amongst the RNA viruses, anywhere from 27 to 32 kilobases. They have their genome protected inside the nucleocapsid, which is further enclosed within a viral envelope with glycoprotein spikes. The spiked envelope comes from their host cell and protects them from the environment while they transfer from host to host. The genome encodes for around five structural proteins, and other associated non-structural proteins. The five structural proteins are: spike (S), membrane (M), envelope (E), nucleocapsid (N), and hemagglutinin-esterase (HE) proteins.

S protein is trimeric and highly N-glycosylated. They generally get cleaved into two functional domains: S1 and S2, by proteases. Here, S1 helps in receptor binding, whereas S2 provides structural support by forming a stalk at the S protein. M protein is important for giving the virion its shape and morphology by accommodating physical bending of the membrane as well as assisting binding to the nucleocapsid. E protein has important functions in the assembly, budding, envelope formation, and pathogenesis of the virus (*Schoeman & Fielding, 2019*). Phosphorylated N protein has more affinity towards the viral RNA genome and binds to it. They ultimately help in packaging by interacting with other related structural and non-structural proteins as well as binding to the genomic packaging signal. HE is exclusive to beta-coronaviruses. They help in viral entry to the host cell by binding to sialic acid and through its esterase activity. It also helps the virus further spread into the host once in the mucosa.

These coronaviruses are zoonotic and lethal in nature as they can cross the species barrier to infect humans. These spillovers increase the chances of novel mutations on top of the inherent genetic instability of the RNA virus. Even with high homology across the other members of the genus, SARS-CoV-2 differs at their S-protein structure from SARS-CoV. They have receptor binding domain (RBD) at S1 which makes close contact with the host Angiotensin-converting enzyme 2 (ACE2) receptor. The RBD has 14 amino acids which directly contact the ACE2 receptor, out of which only conserve 8 are in SARS-CoV-2. While SARS-CoV and SARS-CoV-2 bind to ACE2 receptors in humans, MERS-CoV binds to dipeptidyl-peptidase 4 (DPP4) for viral entry. SARS-CoV however lacks at the furin cleavage site, thus, can only cleave partially. Further, SARS-CoV-2 has 12 extra nucleotides upstream to the cleavage site compared to others. Furin-site facilitates S protein priming by host proteases for viral entry into target cells as well as to accommodate spreading into the host. The specific S protein and receptor interaction determines the tissue selectivity and species specificity of the virus.

SARS-CoV and SARS-CoV-2 have similar genomic organization in the protein coding regions. However, according to S protein and RNA polymerases' phylogenetic study, SARS-CoV-2 is shown as very distant from SARS-CoV. Their S1 domain of S protein has 50 conserved amino acids similarity with closely related RBD. SARS-CoV-2 has 76-78% similarity in spike protein, 73-76% in RBD, and 50-53% sequence similarity in receptor binding motif compared to SARS-CoV. SARS-CoV-2 shares more sequence and structural homology with SARS-CoV than MERS-CoV. SARS-CoV-2 shares the same S protein and manipulates the same proteases for viral entry. (*Rabaan et al., n.d.*)

SARS-CoV-2: Variants of Concern (VOCs) and Variants of Interest (VOIs)

Various criteria are analyzed to decide whether a certain variant is of interest only or of concern that needs close surveillance. Variant-specific genetic marker characterization, prevalence of the variant in a region, its contribution to the increasing cases, etc. are all required to determine VOCs or VOIs. Variants of interest have mutations that have been predicted to have association with enhanced virulence, transmission, diagnostics, therapeutics, or escaping immunity. However, they are not as prevalent around the world to raise concern and do not contribute as much to the peaks of COVID-19 epicurve or result in unique outbreak clusters. VOIs usually do not require any major changes to the existing public health actions as often only a few epidemiological analyses for viral spread or severity, and/ or tighter surveillance etc. would suffice for the unique variant. VOIs become a matter of concern (VOCs) when these variants have evidence for high disease severity, transmission, or negative impact on the available diagnostics, drugs, vaccines, or other therapeutics. Often VOCs have a higher probability of re-infecting individuals immunized by vaccination or primary infection. This brings forth stringent processes to be followed to refrain from a global spread of the VOC in question. By notifying the national level health agency and World Health Organization (WHO), appropriate measures should be taken to contain the spread by putting additional safety controls in place. The VOCs need to be monitored closely by the federal government and characterized to understand its impact on the existing diagnostics and therapeutics. The drugs and vaccines need to be modified or developed accordingly to create a line of defence against these possibly life-threatening VOCs. (*"CDC"*, *2020*)

Variants	Spike Protein mutations	Country of first detection	VOC/VOI	Type of Transmission
B.1.1.7	D614G, P681H, T716I, S982A,Δ69/70, Δ144, N501Y, A570D, D1118H	United Kingdom	VOC	Dominant strain
P.1	D614G, R190S, K417T, E484K, H655Y, T1027I, L18F, T20N, N501Y, P26S, D138Y	Brazil	VOC	Community

Variants	Spike Protein mutations	Country of first detection	VOC/VOI	Type of Transmission
B.1.351	D614G, A701V, K417N, E484K, N501Y, D80A, D215G, Δ241/242/243	South Africa	VOC	Community
B.1.617	D614G, L452R, E484Q	India	VOC	Not Identified Yet
B.1.427	D614G, L452R	United States	VOC	Sporadic
B.1.525	Δ144, D614G, F888L, E484K, A67V, Δ69/70,Q677H,	United Kingdom and Nigeria	VOI	Community
P.2	E484K, D614G, V1176F	Brazil	VOI	Only been detected, is not part of large-scale transmission ye
B.1.526	D614G, T95I, D253G,	United States	VOI	Same as above

("CDC", 2020), ("SARS-CoV-2 variants of concern as of 6 May 2021", n.d.), ("How Many Strains of the Coronavirus Are There? About New Variants", 2021)

Variants that are also strains	Characterization of the behavioral changes	Citations
B.1.1.7	• More infectious and results in a longer infection period without any symptomatic change or in their duration. • Reinfections for this variant is very rare, as immunity from the primary infection would protect against the virus. • More efficient person to person transmission • No impact on susceptibility to emergency use authorization (EUA)* monoclonal antibody treatment • No impact in antibody neutralization by human convalescent or post-vaccination sera	(Davies et al., 2021), (Graham et al., 2021), (Jangra et al., 2021)
P.1	• Reduced susceptibility to combined bamlanivimab and etesevimab monoclonal antibody treatment; however no change in susceptibility to casirivimab with imdevimab combined administration • More resistant to or reduced neutralization by human convalescent plasma or post-vaccination sera	(FACT SHEET FOR HEALTH CARE PROVIDERS EMERGENCY USE AUTHORIZATION (EUA) OF BAMLANIVIMAB AND ETESEVIMAB AUTHORIZED USE, n.d.), (FACT SHEET FOR HEALTH CARE PROVIDERS EMERGENCY USE AUTHORIZATION (EUA) OF REGEN-COV TM (casirivimab with imdevimab), n.d.), (Wang et al., 2021)

Variants that are also strains	Characterization of the behavioral changes	Citations
B.1.351	• Increased infection risk in immunized individuals; greater chance of re-infection • Significant decrease in neutralization by monoclonal antibody: bamlanivimab and etesevimab combined, but no change in susceptibility to casirivimab with imdevimab combined. • Resistance to antibody neutralization by vaccine sera or convalescent plasma.	(Planas et al., 2021), (FACT SHEET FOR HEALTH CARE PROVIDERS EMERGENCY USE AUTHORIZATION (EUA) OF BAMLANIVIMAB AND ETESEVIMAB AUTHORIZED USE, n.d.), (FACT SHEET FOR HEALTH CARE PROVIDERS EMERGENCY USE AUTHORIZATION (EUA) OF REGEN-COV TM (casirivimab with imdevimab), n.d.), (Wang, Liu, et al., 2021)
B.1.617	• Reduced susceptibility to some EUA monoclonal antibody treatments, however, casirivimab with imdevimab to be administered together can effectively fight against the variant. • No impact in sera antibody neutralization obtained from immunized individuals.	(FACT SHEET FOR HEALTH CARE PROVIDERS EMERGENCY USE AUTHORIZATION (EUA) OF BAMLANIVIMAB AND ETESEVIMAB AUTHORIZED USE, n.d.), (FACT SHEET FOR HEALTH CARE PROVIDERS EMERGENCY USE AUTHORIZATION (EUA) OF REGEN-COV TM (casirivimab with imdevimab), n.d.), (Yadav et al., 2021)

EUA monoclonal antibody treatment: FDA authorized bamlanivimab and etesevimab to be administered together for their association with reduced emergency and hospital visits amongst COVID-19 patients mild symptoms with higher risk to severe symptoms and hospitalization. Although the above mentioned is the most used drug combination, there are alternative EUA options: (casirivimab with imdevimab to be administered together, etc. ("An EUA for Bamlanivimab—A Monoclonal Antibody for COVID-19," 2020), (Commissioner, 2021)

What is the likelihood of a mutation to escape immunity? Have SARS-CoV-2 reached there yet?

As ongoing surveillance revealed an enormous number of mutations emerging at the receptor-binding domain of the S protein targeted by many existing vaccines, concerns arise on the emergence of novel variants with the potential of escaping vaccine-mediated immunity due to delay in the delivery of the second dose worldwide.

Current spike protein RBD mutations, such as, K417N/T, E484K, and N501Y, etc. have shown significant reduction in antibody neutralization by vaccinee sera. Resistance towards vaccines is significantly different from escaping existing therapeutics or drugs as vaccines and drugs serve different roles in a patient with COVID-19 infection. Vaccine elicits immune responses to effectively neutralize the virus to prevent any further infections, while drugs try to alleviate the symptoms from an existing infection. Vaccines also target multiple sites to raise immune response against, while drugs focus on fewer sites. Historically, vaccines have been successful in keeping many viral infections in check and extinct in the past. Although minor adjustments have been required to the vaccine for highest efficacy, as seen in influenza vaccines, the need to improve against the viral variations was not driven by the vaccines but because of the natural evolution process. The emergence of resistant variants like B.1.1.7 and B.1.351 increases the probability of such variants emerging by many folds. Adequate research and close monitoring of vaccine delivery and emerging variants are required to get a glimpse of what might vaccine delay mean for the long run. (*Garcia-Beltran et al., 2021*), (*SARS-CoV-2 immunity-escape variants, n.d.*)

Unanswered questions and future directions

As SARS-CoV-2 evolves randomly, they will continue to come up with newer variants. The nature of these variants will determine whether the virus will survive the natural selection. The consequence of the mutation on the virus does not dominate the frequency of a mutation occurring in a generation. For a virus to mutate into any dangerous strain, which adversely affects its human host, is a chance event. It is not necessary that the genotypic change in the variant would result in differences in its behavior. However, if the variant displays behavioral changes, a novel strain is formed. When variants and strains surface, they need to be closely monitored and characterized to understand their association with important areas, such as, disease symptomatology, transmission, immunity, etc. Depending on their characterization, they are categorized as variants of interest (VOI) and variants of concern (VOC). The categorization is not absolute, as the variants may leap between the two classes based on their prevalence amongst the new cases and their contribution in rising to the peak of the transmission curve. These categorizations may differ across the nations due to complete containment of the novel variants locally, amongst other things. Public health measures are required to be adjusted accordingly to contain the spread locally and prevent global transmission. It is important to ensure that the novel variants do not affect the existing diagnostics and therapeutics to achieve a long-lasting immunity against the virus. However, if the variant escapes these vaccines and neutralizing antibody treatments, etc. which is inevitable with the amount of mutations SARS-CoV-2 genome experiences, the drugs and treatments need to be rapidly modified into their next generation for optimal protection.

Chapter 4

Importance of Vaccines during COVID-19

Ida Marchese

COVID-19 Vaccines Protect Oneself and Others

VACCINES TEACH THE immune system to recognize and target various pathogens and create antibodies to fight infection and prevent future infection without contracting the disease itself. Once a person is vaccinated, the new antibodies will aid the immune system in preventing infection and illness. Regarding COVID-19, typically, people infected with the SARS-CoV-2 virus develop an immune response via the production of antibodies due to natural infection. This immune response is generally produced during the first few weeks. The effectiveness of the immune response and the amount of time it lasts is currently under investigation, especially regarding variation in protection across different populations (*"Getting the COVID-19 Vaccine", 2021*).

Therefore, the administration of COVID-19 vaccines results

in an immune response that protects people from infection. This immunity developed via vaccination reduces the risk of contracting COVID-19 and the associated residual health consequences. This immunity via vaccines also aids in fighting the virus if exposed. Thus, vaccination protects oneself in many ways regarding reducing transmission of the SARS-CoV-2 virus and preventing serious illness even if one becomes infected. This is crucial to protect people who are at the highest risk for severe health complications, such as those who are elderly, healthcare providers and those with immunocompromisation and other medical conditions (*"Coronavirus disease (COVID-19): Vaccines"*, 2021).

Suppose a person can get vaccinated. In that case, this will aid in so-called "herd immunity," protecting those who are unable to get vaccinated for various reasons or are at higher risk for infection. Herd immunity results from a large proportion of a population and or community becoming immune to a disease, making transmission from individual to individual less likely. Preventing and lowering the risk of transmission of an illness protects not only those who are immune but also the entire population. If the proportion of the population immune to the disease is more significant than the threshold at which individuals can contract a disease, then the spread of the disease will decline. This phenomenon is known as the herd immunity threshold. In the instance where the proportion of individuals prone to contracting the disease is greater than the proportion of individuals able to become vaccinated and develop immunity, this would lead to an increase in COVID-19 cases despite vaccination. Therefore, it is crucial for public health and safety that every individual eligible and physically able to receive a COVID-19 vaccination must do so to protect those who are unable to obtain a vaccine and lower transmission of infection rates (*"Herd immunity and COVID-19 (coronavirus): What you need to know"*, 2021).

This type of herd immunity via vaccinations is necessary to protect populations and reduce the spread of the virus. Natural immunity and protection via antibodies made by the immune system after a COVID-19 infection are not enough to fully protect individuals as the innate immunity during the initial infection wears off. Furthermore, vaccination is a much safer way to gain protection and limits the possibility of the lasting effects COVID-19 has on a person's health (*"Benefits of Getting a COVID-19 Vaccine", 2021*).

Vaccines and COVID-19 Variants

COVID-19 vaccines were developed based on the SARS-Cov-2 virus before the mutations identified in the variants. Research suggests that against the emerging variants, COVID-19 vaccines have lower efficacy in protecting against infection but still provide protection against acute COVID-19 infection (*"Get the facts about COVID-19 vaccines", 2021*). Current COVID-19 vaccines are expected to provide some degree of protection against variants due to the overall immune response created by the vaccines. Thus the mutations would not result in the current vaccines becoming completely ineffective (*"Coronavirus disease (COVID-19): Vaccines", 2021*). As further research is conducted and data is analyzed, vaccination manufacturers continue to examine whether it is possible to make the vaccine more effectively protect individuals against the different variants (*"Coronavirus disease (COVID-19): Vaccines", 2021*) and develop booster shots to improve protection (*"Get the facts about COVID-19 vaccines", 2021*).

There remains emerging evidence about protection against new variants of the COVID-19 virus. It is important to note that the extent of time and the effectiveness in which fully vaccinated people are protected from variants is uncertain. However, what remains clear is preventing the COVID-19 virus from spreading via transmission and replication, which reduces the risk of the virus mutating and becoming more resistant to vaccines (*"Get the facts about COVID-19 vaccines"*, *2021*).

Maximizing Tools for Pandemic Control

It is important to note that while vaccines are beneficial and a reliable tool to end this pandemic worldwide, society cannot solely rely on vaccines for public health and safety. Considering these unprecedented times and how new COVID-19 is, it is still under investigation how long a person who is vaccinated is protected from infection and whether vaccinated people can still transmit the virus to others (*"Getting the COVID-19 Vaccine"*, *2021*). This is proven further by surges in COVID-19 cases despite the increase in the number of people vaccinated, either fully or partially. While the effects of vaccines on the spread of COVID-19 are still under investigation, wearing proper personal protective equipment (PPE), using reporting and testing services, as well as adhering to government guidelines and protocols are all essential (*"Benefits of Getting a COVID-19 Vaccine"*, *2021*).

Widespread vaccination will aid in the process of getting back to somewhat of a semblance of life pre-pandemic. However, it is essential to note that some things such as increased awareness and concern for public health and safety may become a part of a new normal.

Public and Community Education

The importance of vaccination must be stressed to the public. This can be done in the form of community education. While there is much misinformation about the vaccination process and vaccines themselves, it is vital to make it known that the COVID-19 vaccines work and are safe. There are conflicting views surrounding vaccination, especially in the mainstream media, about whether COVID-19 vaccines help or hinder public health and safety. Through consistent and clear messaging from trusted and reliable sources such as government and regulated healthcare outlets, there is little room for ignorance and deviation away from the scientific basis that grounds vaccine administration and associated benefits. COVID-19 vaccines are safe and effective. To promote transparency and public discourse about the importance of vaccination, continuing to utilize the mechanism for evaluating and regulating the production of vaccines and the public policies of their use will help to ensure that people receive scientifically sound evidence and information (*Schwartz, 2020*).

Inequities in Vaccine Distribution

Despite tremendous public knowledge about the importance of vaccines, there appear to be many inequities and injustices in terms of vaccine distributions. These injustices occur on many levels, including in Canada, North America and worldwide. Many municipalities, especially those in communities with the highest infection rates, received significantly fewer vaccines than other places with minimal spread. In Ontario, Canada it was found that residents living in communities with the lowest COVID-19 infection rates were 1.5 times more likely to have received a vaccine in comparison to Ontarians residing in communities with the highest infection rates (*Mishra et al., 2021*).

Evidence proves that people belonging to marginalized groups are at higher risk of being infected and die from COVID-19. There exist three groups that are disproportionately affected and experience health burdens. These groups include ethnic minorities, socio-economically disadvantaged people, and people who are elderly. This stresses the importance of COVID-19 vaccinations as there continues to be emerging socioeconomic and health impacts brought about by the pandemic that highlights disparities among different communities (*Ali, Asaria & Stranges, 2020*).

Vaccination is one of the main ways to control the COVID-19 pandemic, however a tool is only effective when it is being utilized. Vaccines will only help in preventing infection if they are administered. The importance of the vaccine also relies on the strategic use and administration of those most at risk to prevent further transmission and infection. While many places around the world and Canada are on standby for an influx of vaccines, enough to vaccinate the entirety of the population able to be vaccinated, serving the most impacted and highest risk communities is one of the essential tenets of vaccine importance and distribution. The importance of vaccinations relies heavily on their administration. If vaccines are not distributed strategically to maximize their effectiveness, then importance dwindles as infection rates increase.

Wide variations exist across different countries and among them regarding the distribution of COVID-19 vaccines. While it is expected for some variation to exist due to many circumstances involving policymakers, foreign governing bodies and public officials, there remain issues that threaten global public health. Outbreaks of COVID-19 infection can occur if populations mix where one population achieves a high COVID-19 vaccination rate, and other populations do not (*"Herd immunity and COVID-19 (coronavirus): What you need to know", 2021*).

Minority communities are experiencing a disproportionate burden from COVID-19. The availability of a public health committee authorized vaccines from the Food and Drug Administration (FDA) is the key to improving public health. There remains vaccine hesitancy among groups in these minority communities...This vaccination hesitancy is not consistent and standard among racial and ethnic minority groups; however, due to reasons involving the spread of misinformation which is furthered by inequities and disproportionality in terms of access to vaccines. Community-engaged interventions and learning opportunities are critical to address concerns and support informed decision-making. Proactive and enterprising efforts must continue to be made in terms of vaccination distribution, public education on health and safety, and alleviating the burdens of COVID-19 in these communities. These tenets are paramount of the importance of health equity and justice and further prove the importance of vaccinations (*Webb Hooper, Nápoles & Pérez-Stable, 2021*).

Inequities in vaccine distribution take place also on a global scale. According to WHO Director General Tedros Adhanom Ghebreyesus, in low-income countries on average one in more than five hundred people have received a COVID-19 vaccine whereas in stark contrast in high-income countries about one in four people have received a vaccine (*"Coronavirus: WHO chief criticises 'shocking' global vaccine divide", 2021*). The COVID-19 vaccine purchase data from the Duke Global Health Innovation Center Launch and Scale Speedometer suggests that more than half of all global doses for COVID-19 vaccines have been purchased by high-income countries and estimations suggest that until at least 2023, there will not be enough vaccines for the world's population. Despite high-income countries purchasing more than half of all global vaccine doses, high-income countries represent only a fifth of the global adult population. This results in large disparities between the adult population and the doses for all other country income groups (*"Global COVID-19 Vaccine Access: A Snapshot of Inequality", 2021*).

Global powerhouses such as the USA, United Kingdom, European Union and Japan had secured 1.3 billion doses of vaccines as of August 2020. Countries that are low-income struggle to grapple with the effects of COVID-19 as they are forced into more substantial inequality, and people live in poverty. To ensure fair and equal access to COVID-19 treatments and vaccinations, the Nuffield Council on Bioethics suggests many issues must be addressed. *"These include research funding and priorities, the distribution of burdens and benefits, commercial confidentiality, patents and licensing, pricing, manufacturing and distribution infrastructure, limited supplies and purchasing monopolies, public trust, and distributive justice (Nhamo, Chikodzi, Kunene & Mashula, 2020)"*.

In these instances, there are areas in which nations and global policymakers can collaborate and improve the global approach to addressing COVID-19. These areas include:

"(1) share good practices to stem the further spread of the coronavirus; (2) develop effective vaccines at the earliest possible date; (3) advance preparation for mass production and distribution of anticipated vaccines across the world; (4) assist the most vulnerable nations and territories in fighting the pandemic; (5) manage debt crises and combat famines in developing countries that would have emerged from COVID-19 and; (6) preserve global trade by privileging diversification of supply chains and national strategic reserves over economic nationalism and less efficient forms of production." (*Nhamo, Chikodzi, Kunene & Mashula, 2020*)

Unanswered Questions and Future Directions

While the importance of vaccines, especially during these unprecedented times of COVID-19, is continuously evolving as more scientific revelations are made about COVID-19, and the extent of the effects of different COVID-19 vaccines is explored.

It remains unsure what future vaccinations will look like, how health organizations globally will learn from this experience.

During these extraordinary times of COVID-19, governments all around the world created systems for vaccination distribution. These learning moments will provide opportunities for communities globally to reflect on the different groups that make up their communities and provide opportunities to improve how these communities are served in terms of civic duty, social justice and public health and safety. The COVID-19 pandemic presents an opportunity for creating legislation and regulations that allow for universal access to future vaccinations and treatments, especially during times of crises.

Future will emphasize the cruciality of vaccinations... limiting the number of conspiracy theories not backed by science... hopefully this will also highlight the importance of science-based methodologies and raise public awareness about reliable public information sources and encourage people everywhere to think critically and challenge and research information for themselves...

"reducing the spread of the misinformation through penalties or company interventions, but less so on addressing the underlying concerns of the anti-vaxxer community. The authors suggest that involving anti-vaxxers in the discussion is critical to the acceptance and uptake of the vaccine to COVID-19 when it becomes available" (*Boodoosingh, Olayemi & Sam, 2020*).

Vaccination is an effective way to prevent infection and transmission and develop herd immunity. Among the vaccines developed for COVID-19, many were developed based on prior knowledge and experience with other coronaviruses aiming to induce an immune response involving neutralizing antibodies against viral spike proteins or different receptor binding domains. There remain questions about future scientific challenges for the global health and biomedical community and future directions involving vaccine development (*Chen, 2020*). While the foreseeable future remains uncertain in terms of the direction of the COVID-19 Pandemic, it is essential to highlight the importance of COVID-19 vaccinations and the responsibility of the scientific community to continue to learn more about infection, pathology and epidemiology.

Public confidence and trust in the vaccines are equally as crucial as the vaccines themselves.

Widespread COVID-19 vaccination will be successful only if the belief that vaccines are effective and safe is omnipresent. There must also exist policies that are evidence-based to ensure equitable and prioritized distribution of the vaccines themselves. As the COVID-19 Pandemic continues to impact everyday life for people around the world negatively, the public's trust in tried and accurate scientific methods and expertise is seemingly dwindling among people. However, relying on scientific facts and acting in accordance with public health and safety guidelines proposed by principled government scientists and healthcare experts is the best chance at having COVID-19 vaccines being used to their full potential and protecting communities during this current global health crisis (*Schwartz, 2020*).

The COVID-19 Pandemic is likely only to be under control via an effective distribution and administration process of an effective vaccine. However, many questions still surround vaccine development; however, as expected, vaccine demand has exceeded the first rounds of supply, which adds to the importance of vaccines and their ethical distribution (*Gupta & Morain, 2020*). It remains unclear how long the COVID-19 vaccines will protect COVID-19. Research suggests that against variants of the COVID-19 vaccine, efficacy may be lower. This uncertainty is furthered by mutations leading to new variants which could potentially be more resistant to vaccines (*"Herd immunity and COVID-19 (coronavirus): What you need to know", 2021*). This stresses the importance of vaccination concerning variants...unsure whether new vaccines will be required to help protect people against different variants.

Chapter 5

mRNA Vaccines: Current and Future Perspectives

Terrence Wu

VACCINATION IS A very successful medical breakthrough that has been used in disease prevention and control. Inactivated vaccines are treated using heat and chemicals. Live attenuated vaccines (LAVs) are produced in animal models, cell lines or unfavourable growth conditions (*Zhang et al., 2019*). Protein subunit vaccines contain specifically selected small pieces of the live protein from the original pathogen that are designed to elicit a strong immune response in the patient (*What Are Protein Subunit Vaccines and How Could They Be Used against COVID-19?, n.d.*) A new approach to developing vaccine treatments for infectious diseases is known as messenger RNA (mRNA) vaccines. mRNA vaccines teach our cells to code for a copy of a non-infectious protein that sets out to trigger a strong immune response in the body. Although mRNA vaccines are newer and were developed more recently, they have also been used to combat influenza (flu), Zika, cytomegalovirus (CMV), and rabies (*CDC, 2021*). It is important to clarify that mRNA vaccines are not infectious themselves and will not give the patient the infectious disease. Unlike other vaccination methods, this presents a huge benefit to the design and efficacy of mRNA vaccines, in the sense that patients can gain protection without having to get sick or exposed to the real infectious disease.

Before a vaccine is approved for clinical use, they undergo a stringent series of clinical phases to test for safety and effectiveness. Phase 0 is the pre-clinical trial phase which determines the pharmacodynamics and pharmacokinetics of the drug. Phase I addresses safety concerns. Phase II looks at how effective the drug is at preventing disease. Phase III confirms the safety and efficacy findings from phases I and II. Phase IV looks at sentry studies, while Phase V compares the results from phase III with other drugs that are currently available in the market (*Mahan, 2014*). Regular vaccine development normally takes 10-15 years. However, due to the urgency and increasing demand for therapeutic interventions to alleviate the signs and symptoms of COVID-19, clinical trial phases have been merged together to expedite the process of getting our most vulnerable populations vaccinated against COVID-19 (*Development and Licensure of Vaccines to Prevent COVID-19; Guidance for Industry, n.d.*). The first COVID-19 vaccines were developed within 1.0-1.5 years using an abbreviated clinical trial process. Currently there are two approved mRNA vaccines for preventing the SARS-CoV-2 viral infection. BNT 162b2 from Pfizer-BioNTech and mRNA-1273 by Moderna are two vaccines that teach our body to recognize and fight off the spike (S) protein found on the surface of the SARS-CoV-2 viral capsid shell.

Review Different mRNA Vaccines in Clinical Trials

The BNT 162b2 by Pfizer-BioNTech was approved by Health Canada on December 9, 2020 (*COVID-19 Vaccines for Ontario, n.d.*). The Pfizer vaccine is administered in two 30 µg doses spaced 21 days apart. The results from clinical trials show that it is 95% effective against preventing COVID-19 disease. This vaccine has cleared the mark for having a true vaccine efficacy rate of over 30%, which has exceeded the minimum FDA criteria for authorization (*Polack et al., 2020*).

The mRNA-1273 vaccine by Moderna was approved by Health Canada on December 23, 2020 (*COVID-19 Vaccines for Ontario, n.d.*). The mRNA vaccine shows the immune system what the SARS-CoV-2 spike (S) protein looks like, so it can build its own defenses against the virus. This trial took place in the United States of America and the participants included 45 healthy adults who received two vaccinations 28 days apart. The participants either received a dose of 25µg, 100µg, or 250µg. After the first vaccination, there were more antibodies in larger doses. After the second vaccination, the antibody titer levels were higher. More than half of the participants experienced fatigue, chills, headaches, muscle pain, and general inflammation. The participants who received a higher dosage reported at least one of the severe adverse events. The mRNA-1273 vaccine is effective against suppressing the pathogenesis and transmission of the SARS-CoV-2 (*L. A. Jackson et al., 2020*).

CVnCoV is a vaccine produced by CureVac. At the time of writing, this vaccine has not yet been approved for clinical use. However, it is currently undergoing Phase 2b/3 clinical trials which were initiated in mid-December 2020. Similar to Pfizer and Moderna's mRNA vaccines, CureVac uses a full-length spike protein with the amino acid, proline substituted within the mRNA transcript. The genome is placed inside an ionizable cationic lipid nanoparticle. It is administered intramuscularly with 2 doses spaced 28 days apart (*Verbeke et al., 2021*).

Safety and Effectiveness of mRNA vaccines

Vaccines can be delivered through non-viral, nucleic acid-based mechanisms. Large manufacturing chains of these vaccine agents are safer and more time-saving than working with live infectious reagents, which have a much larger chance for releasing dangerous pathogens into the environment (*Zhang et al., 2019*). The manufacturing process of mRNA vaccines does not use toxic chemicals or pathogenic cell cultures, unlike some other vaccine platforms, including live viral vectors, attenuated viruses, inactivated viruses, and subunit protein vaccines (*Pardi et al., 2018*).

A part of why the mRNA vaccines are so successful is because of the use of nanomedicine drug delivery systems. This is a non-viral delivery mechanism that is not raised as a red flag to the immune system. Through multiple rounds of clinical trials and testing phases, lipid nanoparticle mRNA vaccines have a 95% efficacy rate and many of these vaccines have earned FDA approval (*Kim et al., 2021*). It carries the genetic information and releases into the muscles. The white blood cells read the information from the mRNA and alerts the other immune cells. This starts the process to start building host defences against SARS-CoV-2, specifically the spike protein. The lipid nanoparticle that carries the genetic information is easily processed by the body (*Buschmann et al., 2021*). The process for making nanomedicines is through microfluidic mixing and controlling for a low pH environment to protonate the amine function of the ionizable lipid. It is important to balance the electrostatic relationships between the positively-charged lipid particles and the negatively-charged mRNA to develop a stable structure to withhold the densely packed mRNA (*Verbeke et al., 2021*).

So far, the results gathered from clinical trials has shown that the Pfizer and Moderna vaccines have had no serious side effects that resulted in patients being hospitalized (*Krammer et al., 2021*). However, there are some side effects associated with mRNA vaccinations. The most common side effects surround the localized site of injection. These signs could include, but are not limited to, inflammation, pain and swelling (*Krammer et al., 2021*).

Different Ways of Building mRNA Vaccines

mRNA vaccines are much easier and quicker to synthesize in the laboratory, where mRNA products can be produced in high amounts. They can also be transported and stored more readily than traditional live attenuated or inactivated vaccines, which primarily consist of protein-based vaccines (*Zeng et al., 2020*).

There are two types of mRNA vaccine platforms that can be used to deliver the targeted genomic transcript of an immunogen. There are a few commonalities between both mRNA constructs, which include similar cap structures, 5' and 3' untranslated regions (UTRs), open-reading frames (ORFs), and a 3' poly-A tail (*Pardi et al., 2018*). Non-replicating mRNA (NRM) encodes the coding sequence of the targeted protein to be made. Self-amplifying mRNA (SAM) includes genetic replication machinery commonly found in positive-stranded mRNA alphaviruses. The genetic information produced by NRMs and SAMs are translated by ribosomes, which is followed by post-translational modifications. Both of these constructs can be formed in lipid nanoparticles for better structure, stabilization, prevent degradation and promote cellular uptake (*N. A. C. Jackson et al., 2020*).

Vaccine Supply and Storage

Many mRNA vaccines have a limited shelf-life, as they need to be kept at very low temperatures. Current research is now looking into making these mRNA vaccines more structurally stable and less resistant to environmental damage. mRNA vaccines need to be successfully screened and purified to remove contaminants that may affect their efficacy ratings. Some mRNA platforms need to be purified and placed into a sterile storage buffer before being allocated and shipped in vials for clinical use and administration (*Pardi et al., 2018*).

Due to the delicate chemical structure of mRNA, most mRNA

products are currently stored frozen at -70°C or -94°F. This presents a critical limitation to delivering and administering vaccines to developing countries, where the technology may not be available to support proper vaccine distribution (*Pardi et al., 2018*). The chemical stability of the mRNA is impacted by the colloidal stability of the vaccine products (*Crommelin et al., 2021*). Researchers have looked into embedding mRNA vaccines into nucleic acid-based macromolecules (NAM) to improve the stability of the mRNA in non-viral systems (*Muralidhara et al., 2016*). Studies have also been done on freeze-drying naked mRNA to improve their structural strength before being placed into vials. The freeze-dried formulation is stable enough to be stored at temperatures ranging from -80°C to +70°C or -112°F to +158°F (*Jones et al., 2018*). There are also analytical methods that can be used to measure mRNA vaccine stability, which look at the identity, purity, potency, safety, and stability of the mRNA lipid-protein complex (*Poveda et al., 2019*).

Vaccine Administration and Delivery

There are many routes of administration for mRNA vaccine delivery, including intradermal injection, subcutaneous injection, intravenous injection, and intranodal injection (*Zeng et al., 2020*). Intranasal sprays are currently being developed for COVID-19 vaccinations. BBV154 is a novel adenovirus-vectored vaccine developed by Bharat Biotech. This vaccine is delivered through the nasal pathway to elicit broad immune responses to COVID-19, including neutralizing immunoglobulin G (IgG), mucosal immunoglobulin A (IgA), and T-lymphocyte cell responses (*Hassan et al., 2020*).

Many mRNA vaccines, including those developed by Pfizer and Moderna, are currently injected at an intramuscular site (usually in the muscle of the upper arm) (*Verbeke et al., 2021*). There are delivery vectors that can be used to help the targeted mRNA sequences enter the host cells for recognition and processing (*Kim et al., 2021*). Many mRNA vaccines are built through the process of self-assembly. This process is driven by non-covalent interactions, which use the random and spontaneous arrangement of different molecules to form a supramolecular assembly (*Bishop et al., 2009*).

Vaccines can also be stored in other delivery carriers, including lipid nanoparticles, polymers, peptides, free mRNA in solution and ex vivo through dendritic cells (*Zeng et al., 2020*). Lipid-based nanoparticles are typically prepared using continuous-flow microfluidic devices which are used in vivo for rapid diffusion and polarity changes during the self-assembled formation of the mRNA-lipid nanoparticle complex (Arteta et al., 2018). Vaccines can also be administered via polymer-based delivery mechanisms. This classification represents a group of functional materials, including polyamines, dendrimers, and copolymers, which have the machinery capable of delivering mRNA vaccines. The caveat with using polymer-based mechanisms is that they have limited stability levels. This can be improved by attaching lipid chains, hyperbranched groups and biodegradable subunits (*Dong et al., 2016; Kaczmarek et al., 2016; Patel et al., 2019*). When peptides are used for vaccine delivery, they are usually positively-charged which allows these molecules to interact with nucleic acids through electrostatic interactions (*Zeng et al., 2020*). During the early development of mRNA vaccines, protamine was a commonly used cationic peptide. Protamine has protective features which prevents mRNA degradation, improving overall vaccine stability (*Hoerr et al., 2000*). Protamine peptides have also been shown to be very beneficial in protecting the mRNA from harsh storage conditions, which affects the safety and efficacy of the vaccine, as mentioned earlier (*Stitz et al., 2017*). Free mRNA can be co-delivered with other antigen formulations, making this type of vaccine delivery platform applicable for building immunity against many types of viral infections and cancers (*Zeng et al., 2020*).

Application of mRNA vaccines - Oncolytic viral therapy

Modern vaccination approaches can be applied and designed for non-infectious diseases, including cancer (*Pardi et al., 2018*). Oncolytic virus therapy is becoming a larger and more popular field in vaccination research. Different viruses can be slightly modified using genetically engineered viral vectors to be applied as a therapeutic intervention for cancer patients. Selected oncolytic viruses have high selectivity to kill targeted cancerous cells to stop and prevent their proliferation in forming tumours in the tissues and organs of the human body (*Fukuhara et al., 2016; Yaghchi et al., 2015*).

In modern times, animal viruses are now able to be genetically engineered based on our current knowledge and understanding of viral replication (*Palese, 1998*). There are many advantages to using RNA-based viral vectors. That they have good in vitro applications in cell culture studies and the proteins can be expressed at very high levels making them excellent vaccine delivery platforms. There are also no infectious viral particles produced, reducing viral spreading and transmission. Another advantage is that, since these genetically engineered viruses do not contain the original structural proteins found in the live virus, the strength of the host immune response is limited making this a great opportunity to build innate and adaptive host defence mechanisms to various types of pathogens. By understanding the viral life cycle, researchers know that RNA doesn't readily incorporate into chromosomal DNA which removes the possibility of unwanted integration of genomic information into the host cells by mistake (*Agapov et al., 1998*).

Unanswered Questions and Future Directions

Further research is needed to determine whether existing vaccines become less effective due to pre-existing immunity to viral agents. Immunosuppression can be used to determine where tumours are located within the body, in order to direct the vaccine therapy to the right location within the body. There is also a question of how different animal models are used in clinical trials to test the safety and effectiveness of the components of mRNA vaccines. It is well understood that as there are physiological differences between animal models and humans, there will be some discrepancies to how inflammatory signals and immune signalling pathways work to combat disease. There are still barriers associated with making vaccines more successful at overcoming the strong immune responses coming from the adaptive immune system. Future directions should examine how to best support ongoing scientific initiatives in developing sustainable and effective therapies for infectious diseases to prevent the onset of future pandemics.

The development of mRNA vaccines presents an innovative breakthrough that is made possible due to the capabilities of modern science. Vaccination is a very successful and useful tool that can be used to treat and prevent a wide range of infectious diseases. It also has many clinical applications, including onco-lytic virology and cancer therapies.

Chapter 6

Pfizer-BioNTech Vaccine

Cynthia Xu

CREATED BY PFIZER and BioNTech, tozinameran (or BNT162b2) was one of the first widely approved mRNA vaccines for COVID-19. Formulated in a lipid nanoparticle (LNP) composition, BNT162b2 is a nucleoside-modified mRNA (modRNA) vaccine that encodes for a SARS-CoV-2 spike glycoprotein. By presenting the body with a small portion of the viral sequence contained in SARS-CoV-2, the body produces the spike protein displayed on the surface of the virus. That spike protein is what generates an immune response to the virus to potentially prevent infection (*Pfizer, 2020*).

Having been authorized in Canada on December 9, 2020, it is currently available for people who are 12 years of age or older. Like other COVID-19 vaccines however, the safety and effectiveness of the vaccine for people under 16 years of age is still under evaluation and not well established. Similar to most vaccines, the tozinameran is given by a 0.3 mL dose injection into the muscle of the arm and takes about two weeks to develop significant production against COVID-19. In order to reach full effectiveness however, a second dose is required 21 days after the first (*Government of Canada, 2021*).

Side Effects

Like with all vaccines, there is risk for some side effects. The most commonly reported side effects in the clinical trials were mild or moderate and consisted of: pain at the site of injection, chills, tiredness, headache, muscle pain, joint pain and fever. These were found to be more common in people who were getting a second dose rather than their first (*U.S. Food & Drug Administration, 2021*). Serious side effects are extremely rare and result due to severe allergic reactions to the vaccine. Health Canada has conducted a scientific review of the available medical evidence and continues to do so to assess the safety of the Pfizer-BioNTech COVID-19 vaccine. As of current state, no major safety concerns have been identified (*Government of Canada, 2021*).

Efficacy

Among 36 523 participants who had no evidence of existing or prior SARS-CoV-2 infection, 8 cases of COVID-19 were observed in vaccine recipients who had their second dose at least seven days prior. With COVID-19 being presented in 162 placebo recipients, this case split corresponds to 95.0% vaccine efficacy. Among all the participants, including those with evidence of prior SARS CoV-2 infection, 9 cases of COVID-19 at least seven days after the second dose were observed among BNT162b2 recipients and 169 in the placebo group. This results in the corresponding vaccine efficacy of 94.6%. Furthermore, similar vaccine efficacy was observed across subgroups defined by age, sex, race, ethnicity, baseline body-mass index (BMI), and the presence of coexisting conditions.

While all these efficacy studies were taken at least a week after the second dose, between the first and second dose, 39 cases in the BNT162b2 group and 82 cases in the placebo group were observed. Thus, resulting in a vaccine efficacy of 52%. This indicates that early protection by the vaccine starts as soon as

12 days after the first dose (*Polack et al., 2020*).

Trials

Conducted in Germany and the United States, BioNTech and Pfizer initially launched a coordinated program to compare four RNA-based COVID-19 vaccine candidates in umbrella-type clinical studies. The program was designed to support the selection of a single vaccine candidate and dose level for an international safety and efficacy trial. Based on the initial clinical trial results in Germany, two LNP formulated, nucleoside modRNA vaccine candidates for SARS-CoV-2 were selected to be evaluated in the phase 1 portion of the trial in the United States, BNT162b1 and BNT162b2. BNT162b1, encodes the SARS-CoV-2 receptor-binding domain, trimerized by the addition of a T4 fibritin foldon domain to increase its immunogenicity through multivalent display. BNT162b2, on the other hand, encodes the SARS-CoV-2 full-length spike, modified by two proline mutations to lock in the perfusion conformation and more closely mimic the intact virus with which the elicited virus-neutralizing antibodies must interact (*Walsh et al., 2020*).

Phase 1

In a randomized, placebo-controlled, observer-blinded, dose-escalation trial, the purpose of phase 1 was to select the final vaccine candidate and a dose level. The two vaccine candidates, BNT162b1 and BNT162b2, were given on a 2-dose schedule (separated by 21 days) at 10 µg, 20 µg or 30 µg dose levels and were then evaluated for their active immunization against COVID-19. There was also one group of participants aged 18 to 55 who was assigned to receive one 100 µg dose of BNT162b1 or placebo (*Pfizer, 2020*). All vaccine candidates were administered through an intramuscular injection to the deltoid muscle.

Each group studied in phase 1 consisted of 15 healthy participants, with 3 of them receiving placebos. This surmounted to a total of 13 groups and 195 participants and the participants' ages were classified into 18 to 55 years of age or 65 to 85 years of age. Prior to the vaccinations, the participants were all screened based on a set list of criteria, with the key exclusion being: having a known infection with a human immunodeficiency virus; an immunocompromised condition; a history of autoimmune disease; a previous diagnosis of COVID-19; pregnant or breastfeeding; a positive test for SARS-CoV-2 immunoglobulin M (IgM) and/or immunoglobulin G (IgG) antibodies at the screening visit; and positive nasal-swab results on a SARS-CoV-2 nucleic acid amplification test within 24 hours before the receipt of the trial vaccine or placebo.

To ensure safety, for the first vaccine candidate, age group or dose level, the first five participants were observed by blinded site staff for at least 4 hours after vaccination for any acute reactions and the vaccination of the remaining participants started no sooner than 24 hours after the fifth participant received his or her vaccination (*Pfizer, 2020*). All the other participants were observed for 30 minutes and blood samples were collected for safety and immunogenicity assessments (*Walsh et al., 2020*). The decision to escalate to the next dose level was based on a review of the 7 day (minimum) post-dose safety data and the group of participants aged 65 to 85 did not start receiving vaccines until the safety data for the RNA platform had been deemed acceptable at the same, or a higher, dose level in the 18 to 55 year cohort (*Pfizer, 2020*).

Within seven days after injection, participants who received 10 µg, 20 µg, or 30 µg of BNT162b1, reported mild to moderate local reactions (pain at injection site, redness and swelling). Pain at the injection site was the most frequently reported instance and these local reactions were found to be more frequent after the second dose. A similar pattern was observed after vaccination with BNT162b2, with the only difference being that no older participant who received BNT162b2 reported redness or swelling.

In terms of systemic events, participants aged 18 to 55 who received 10 μg, 20 μg, or 30 μg of BNT162b1 frequently had mild to moderate fever and chills, with 75% of the participants reporting a temperature of 38.00C or higher after the second 30 μg dose. In participants 65 to 85 years old, systemic events due to BNT162b1 injection were milder, with 33% reporting a temperature of 38.00C or higher after the second dose. Despite this, many older participants reported fatigue and headache however and one participant reported a fever of 38.9 to 40.00C. Like local reactions, systemic events were greater after the second dose than the first and generally resolved by day 7. Systemic events in response to BNT162b2 were milder than those in response to BNT162b1, with 17% of participants aged 18 to 55 and 8% of those 65 to 85 years of age reporting a fever after the second dose. Severe systemic events (fatigue, headache, chills, muscle pain, and joint pain) were also reported in a smaller number of younger recipients and no severe systemic events were reported by older recipients.

It is also worthy to note that no participant who received either vaccine candidate reported a severe, life-threatening, local reaction or systemic event. After a month of receiving the second dose, 50% of participants aged 18 to 55 who received 30 μg of BNT162b1 reported adverse effects, while participants aged 65 to 85 reported 17%. For BNT162b2 however, only 25% of participants aged 18 to 55 reported adverse effects, with the older recipients reporting none.

The serologic responses elicited by the two candidates were similar and the antigen-binding IgG and virus-neutralizing responses to vaccination with 10 μg to 30 μg of BNT162b1 or BNT162b2 were found to be boosted by the second dose. Higher doses were shown to elicit somewhat higher antibody responses.

Due to BNT162b2 being associated with a lower incidence and severity of systemic reactions than BNT162b1, BNT162b2 at the 30 μg dose level was selected to progress to phase 2-3, international trial (*Welsh et al., 2020*).

Phase 2/3

Phase 2/3 was a multinational, placebo-controlled, observer-blinded efficacy trial that consisted of 43 548 participants aged 16 and up, across six different countries (United States, Argentina, Brazil, South Africa, Germany and Turkey). The number of participants who received a placebo was randomized in a 1:1 ratio and the dosing procedure was the same as phase 1 (two doses, 21 days apart).

In order for the phase 2/3 study population to be as representative and as diverse as possible, participants with known chronic stable HIV diseases were also included. People who had a medical history of COVID-19, treatment with immunosuppressive therapy, or diagnosed with an immunocompromising condition were still excluded however.

Similar to what was seen during the phase 1 trials, most BNT162b2 recipients reported mild to moderate pain at the injection site within 7 days after an injection. A noticeably lower percentage of participants reported redness or swelling however and the proportion of participants reporting local reactions did not increase after the second dose. These mild to moderate reactions were generally resolved in 1 to 2 days. Additionally, results also showed that less than 1% of participants reported severe pain and no participant reported a severe, life-threatening local reaction.

For systemic events, like in phase 1, effects were reported more often by younger vaccine recipients (16 to 55 years of age) than by the older participants (older than 55) and were reported more frequently after dose 2 than dose 1. The most commonly reported systemic events were fatigue and headache, with the frequency of any severe systemic event after the first dose being 0.9%. Severe systemic events were reported in less than 2% of vaccine recipients after either dose, except for fatigue (in 3.8%) and headache (in 2.0%) after the second dose. A fever above 380C was reported within the first 1 to 2 days after the second dose by 16% of younger vaccine recipients and by 11% of older recipients. These symptoms resolved shortly thereafter.

When studying adverse events in 43 252 participants, 27% and 17% of BNT162b2 recipients and placebo recipients reported an adverse event, respectively. 0.3% of vaccine recipients and <0.1% of placebo recipients reported lymphadenopathy and four serious adverse events were reported among BNT162b2 recipients (shoulder injury related to vaccine administration, right axillary lymphadenopathy, paroxysmal ventricular arrhythmia, and right leg paresthesia). Two BNT162b2 recipients died (one from arteriosclerosis and one from cardiac arrest), as did four placebo recipients (two from unknown causes, one from hemorrhagic stroke and one from myocardial infarction). None of these deaths were considered to be related to the vaccine or placebo however and no COVID-19-associated deaths were observed (*Polack et al., 2020*). Pfizer plans to continue to monitor all their participants for up to two years after they received their second dose (*Pfizer, 2020*).

In continuation of the phase 3 study, Pfizer expanded their participant pool to include adolescents aged 12 to 15. Consisting of 2 260 participants, BNT162b2 demonstrated 100% efficacy and robust antibody responses, exceeding those reported in vaccinated 16 to 25 year olds participants in a previous analysis. The side effects were described as well tolerated as well, and were similar to those observed in past phase 2/3 studies for 16 to 55 year olds.

Future Directions and Unanswered Questions

Currently, Pfizer and BioNTech are evaluating the safety, tolerability and immunogenicity of the BNT162b2 vaccine in children 6 months to 11 years of age. Like the previous phases, they are being evaluated on a two-dose schedule, approximately 21 days apart, and are separated in three age groups: 5 to 11 years, 2 to 5 years, and 6 months to 2 years (*Pfizer Inc., 2021 a*).

Pfizer is also evaluating the vaccine's ability to prevent COVID-19 in healthy pregnant women aged 18 and older. The trial will consist of approximately 4 000 individuals who will be vaccinated during 24 to 34 weeks of gestation using the same procedure as the past phase trials. Each woman will participate in the study for approximately seven to ten months and will help assess the safety in infants of vaccinated pregnant women and the potential transfer of protective antibodies to their offspring. The infants will be monitored till they are approximately six months of age (*Pfizer Inc., 2021 b*).

Taking the ongoing studies into account, questions surrounding the potential long term effects still remain. Despite Pfizer stating that it will be monitoring their participants for up to two years after their second vaccine dose, not much is known about their timeline after that. It is also unknown if Pfizer and BioNTech plan to expand their age pool further and include infants younger than 6 months as well as elders older than 85.

Conclusions

Overall, the Pfizer-BioNTech COVID-19 vaccine has made great strides in the mRNA vaccine field and has played a pivotal role in combating the global pandemic. Following phase 1 of the clinical trials, BNT162b2 was chosen over BNT162b1 to proceed to phase 2/3 (*Welsh et al., 2020*). In phase 2/3, the BNT162b2 vaccine was tested on approximately 44 000 participants, ranging from ages 12 to 85 and the safety, tolerability and immunogenicity was noted. BNT162b2 proved to be effective at preventing COVID-19, with a vaccine efficacy of 95% and showed mild to moderate side effects (*Polack et al., 2020*). With it being one of the first vaccines to receive approval for adolescents 12 to 15 years of age, BNT162b2 will be a key component in helping students return to school and bringing the younger generation back to normality.

Chapter 7

Moderna Vaccine - Suhel

Suhel Sadik Patel

About Moderna

MODERNA, INC. WAS founded in 2010 and is currently head-quartered in Cambridge, Massachusetts. It has been named a top biopharmaceutical employer by Science for the past five years. Moderna, Inc. is trying to be the first to engineer a new class of medicine designed with mRNA. The therapeutic areas of focus for these new generations of transformative medicine included areas such as autoimmune diseases, immuno-oncology, cardiovascular diseases, rare diseases and infectious diseases. They currently have 24 development programs that have entered the pipeline with 13 having entered clinical studies. (*Moderna, Inc, 2021*) In addition to their success with their COVID-19 mRNA-1273 vaccine, other advancements in preclinical development with potential to prevent diseases such as Cytomegalovirus (CMV), solid tumors/lymphomas, Myocardial ischemia, and personalized cancer vaccine (PCV) which utilizes mRNA-4157 have also had quite a success. Some notable partners of Moderna, Inc include AstraZeneca, Darpa, and Bill and Melinda Gates Foundation (*Moderna, Inc, 2021*).

How SARS-CoV-2 Works?

In order to understand how the Moderna COVID-19 vaccine works, or for that sense, any COVID-19 vaccine, it is first important to understand how SARS-CoV-2 works to evade our bodies immune system and cause the COVID-19 disease. The SARS-CoV-2 virus has S spike proteins which help it to attach to cell surfaces. The ACE2 receptor is a molecule that is found on the surface of human arterial and venous endothelial cells and arterial smooth muscle cells of organs including the lungs, heart, liver and kidney. The ACE2 receptor is a key landing site of the spike protein found on the surface of SARS-CoV-2 allowing it to attach to cells and undergo structural changes which enable it to fuse with the host cell. Once inside the host cell, the virus particle is uncoated and the virus genome is able to enter the host cytoplasm. SARS-CoV-2 has a single copy of a single stranded positive configuration genome (+ssRNA). The uncoated genome (+ssRNA) is able to overtake the host's own replication machinery, mainly the host cell's ribosomes, and begin producing proteins. Since, +ssRNA is in the same configuration as host cells mRNA, it can begin translation of their proteins directly in the cytoplasm. The proteins made will consist of RNA polymerases and structural components (late phase proteins) of the virus. In the golgi apparatus of the host cells, the proteins will be packaged up with a copy of +ssRNA, forming new replicated viruses. These new viruses will move into secretory vesicles and release into the extracellular environment where it can infect neighbouring health cells and can also be released as respiratory droplets to the surrounding environment. Through this entire process of virus replication, the virus is able to invade host immune recognition, as interferon production is significantly reduced and/or delayed and the innate immune system response is impaire and incapable of recognizing SARS-CoV-2 virus before it is too late. Understanding this, it can help us understand that if we can generate a pseudo SARS-CoV-2 trigger in the human body, the host adaptive immune system can generate an antibody response to the pseudo stimulus. Since, the adaptive immune system is capable of immunological memory, in future encounters of real SARS-CoV-2, the immune system is prepared with pre-formed antibodies capable of recognizing virus associated molecules allowing it it to initiate a response before the virus can attach to host cells or overtake cytoplasmic replication machinery. mRNA vaccines, such as the Moderna and Pfizer- BioNtech COVID-19 vaccine, serve as this pseudo SARS-CoV-2 trigger/stimulus to generate antibodies in the host allowing it to prepared for adaptive recognition when encountering the real virus before it can cause infection and damage to host cells.

What is in the Moderna COVID-19 Vaccine and How Does it Work?

The Moderna COVID-19 vaccine, also called mRNA-1273 is manufactured by ModernaTX, Inc. It is administered in an attempt to prevent COVID-19. Similar to other vaccines authorized in Canada, it is an mRNA vaccine and it is administered to the muscle of the upper arm (*Government of Canada, 2021*). mRNA-1273 is an mRNA-based vaccine made up of a novel lipid nanoparticle (LNP)-encapsulated mRNA. The mRNA encodes a full length and stabilized spike protein of SARS-CoV-2 (*CDC, 2021*). This spike protein created by human ribosomes using the mRNA administered in the vaccine, induces immune response resulting in antibody generation, without the adverse side effects that would occur under SARS-CoV-2 virus exposure. When individuals who are vaccinated and whose immune systems have generated an adequate antibody immune response encounter the live virus, their bodies are prepared to recognize and attack the foreign virus before it gets a chance to infect their cells and induce the unpleasurable, potentially severe, and sometimes life threatening symptoms associated with COVID-19. Currently, the Moderna COVID-19 vaccine has been approved for individuals under the age of 18, however in younger people, safety and effectiveness has not been established. Health Canada authorized this vaccine on December 23, 2020 (*Government of Canada, 2021*).

Vaccine Efficacy

Data from clinical trials conducted with the Moderna COVID-19 vaccine demonstrated that in people who received two doses of the vaccine and had no previous exposure to the virus, it is 94.1% effective at preventing laboratory-confirmed COVID-19 disease (*Moderna, Inc, 2021*). Similar effectiveness was also observed among the diverse population pool included in the clinical trials regardless or age, sex, ethnicity, race and people with a variety of underlying medical conditions who were at an occupational risk to exposure.

Phase I Clinical Trial

The purpose of this clinical trial was to study the safety, reactogenicity and immunogenicity of 2019-nCoV vaccine (mRNA-1273) for prophylaxis of SARS-CoV-2 Infection (COVID-19). Phase I clinical trials for the Moderna COVID-19 vaccine began on March 16, 2020 (*Moderna, Inc, 2021*). This phase I trial was open-label since both the healthcare providers and patients were aware of the treatment being administered and the study was also dose-ranging (*Moderna, Inc, 2021*). Inclusion criteria determined for study participants were stringent, some notable criteria include but are not limited to; age (18-55 years old), males, non-pregnant females, and individuals were required to be in good health as determined by a medical history and physical examination (*FDA, 2020*) (*NIAID, 2020*).

The results from this first phase were quite successful in eliciting an immune response of adequate magnitude. Immunogenicity data demonstrated that dose-dependent increases in immuno-genicity were observed across three dose levels (25µg, 100µg, and 250µg) (*Moderna, Inc, 2021*). Two weeks post administration of the second 25µg dose, the levels of binding antibodies seen in the vaccinated individuals were similar to and at the level of those seen in the blood of patients that had recovered from COVID-19. In addition, two weeks post-administration of the second dose of the 100µg dose, in the 10 participants included in this cohort, they observed significantly higher levels of binding antibodies in the serum compared to the levels seen in the serum of patients that recovered from COVID-19 (*Moderna, Inc, 2021*).

Furthermore, they concluded based on phase I trial data, that the mRNA-1273 used in the Moderna COVID-19 vaccine was generally safe and well tolerated. However, it was not completely clear of any adverse side effects. One participant in the 100µg cohort experienced grade 3 systemic systems consisting of erythema at the site of injection. At this time, the most severe systemic symptoms were observed in 3 participants of the 250µg cohort, but they were only noted after the second dose and all symptoms were transient and self-resolving (*Moderna, Inc, 2021*). Fortunately, grade 4 symptoms or any serious symptoms were reported, which justified further grounds for moving the clinical trials for the mRNA-1273 Moderna COVID-19 vaccine to phase II trials. However, based on the safety reports seen with receiving the 250µg dose, the second phase of this clinical trial was amended to include only 25µg and 100µg doses (*Moderna, Inc, 2021*).

Phase II Clinical Trial

Based on the results and data from phase I clinical studies, Moderna Inc. was granted a Fast Track Designation by the FDA for mRNA-1273 on May 12, 2020 (*Moderna, Inc, 2021*). This allowed them to proceed to phase II of the study in mid-late May. The purpose of the phase II study was to study the safety and immunogenicity of the mRNA-1273 COVID-19 vaccine. 600 participants were enrolled. It was a randomized, observed-blinded, placebo-controlled, dose-confirmation study, with two doses, 50µg and 100µg, as deemed appropriate based on phase I clinical data (*Moderna, Inc, 2021*).

Phase III Clinical Trial

Phase III of the Moderna COVID-19 study was a Coronavirus Efficacy and Safety Study (COVE Study). This study was a randomized, starified, observer-blind, placebo controlled design and included 30,418 participants. Only 100µg was administered following a two-dose regime and the doses were timed 28 days apart (*Moderna, Inc, 2021*). Two endpoints were decided to base analyses upon, the first endpoint analysis was two weeks post-second dose administration and the secondary endpoint analysis analyzed severe cases of COVID-19.

Safety Data

The primary analysis included 196 COVID-19 cases, 11 of these cases were observed in individuals in the Moderna COVID-19 vaccine cohort and 185 of these cases were seen in the placebo group (*Moderna, Inc, 2021*). This demonstrated a strong vaccine efficacy of 94.1% (*CDC, 2021*). The purpose of the secondary analysis was to study severe cases of COVID-19. It included 30 severe cases, and every single one was found in the placebo cohort, no severe cases were observed in the Moderna COVID-19 vaccinated cohort. Additionally, in the placebo group, there was one COVID-19 associated death, and no COVID-19 associated deaths were seen in the vaccine cohort groups (*Moderna, Inc, 2021*). These are quite successful results as they demonstrated not only good efficacy but also good safety and tolerance with a large sample size. Based on a November 25, 2020 cut-off date established for the phase III clinical trial, they were able to gather 9 weeks of safety data post-second dose which set the baseline safety dataset.

Most Notable Side Effects

Injection site pain was the most common adverse experienced by recipients of the two doses of the Moderna COVID-19 vaccine. Additionally, headaches, fatigue, and myalgia were all reactions that were more common in the vaccinated cohort compared to the placebo group (*CDC, 2021*). 2.9% of the total adverse reactions seen, which were classified as severe, were observed after the first dose, and 15.8% of these were after the second dose. Fortunately, the majority of these local adverse reactions were short lived with a median persistence of one to two days (*Moderna, Inc, 2021*) (*FDA, 2021*).

Demographic Information

A major strength of this clinical study was the use of a large sample size (n = 30,418) (*FDA, 2021*). In addition, randomization and the broad demographic characteristics, reflecting the general population, of the participants included in the study increased strength and wide applicability of the vaccine results. The mean age of the participants was 51.6 years ± 15.50, 47.4% female and 52.6% were male (*FDA, 2021*). Sex, ethnicity, age and other demographic data were evenly distributed between the placebo and vaccinated groups. 25.3% of individuals were over the age of 65 (*FDA, 2021*).

In addition to the large sample size, one key difference between the inclusion criteria of the phase I clinical trial and phase III clinical trials was the inclusion of participants with prior diseases or conditions, in the latter, that put them at an increased risk of severe COVID-19 diseases. These conditions included high-risk chronic diseases such as Diabetes (Type 1, Type 2, or gestational), severe obesity (body mass index > 40kg/m2), significant cardiac disease (e.g., heart failure, coronary artery disease, congenital heart disease, cardiomyopathies, and pulmonary hypertension), chronic lung disease (e.g., emphysema and chronic bronchitis, idiopathic fibrosis, and cystic fibrosis), liver disease, human immunodeficiency virus (HIV) infection, and moderate or severe asthma (*FDA, 2021*). Age and health risks associated with severe COVID-19 symptoms were used as stratification factors for randomization (*FDA, 2021*). However, immunocompromised individuals and people with prior COVID-19 infection were excluded from the study (*FDA, 2021*). Determination of previous COVID-19 infection was established through an antibody serum test for antibodies against the SARS-CoV-2 surface proteins.

Conclusion

The Moderna mRNA-1273 COVID-19 vaccine has been approved for use in Canada, United States, Sweden, United Kingdom, Israel, Qatar, Singapore and other countries in Europe (*Moderna, Inc, 2021*).

The use of the Moderna mRNA-1273 COVID-19 vaccine in preventing coronavirus disease 2019 has been demonstrated to be safe and effective through well established clinical studies. However, the work is not complete, phase III of the clinical trials is still ongoing and will follow participants for two years post-second dose of the vaccine. This extended follow-up period after the two-dose series will help scientists, physicians, and law makers determine the long term safety, duration of effectiveness in preventing against COVID-19 and effectiveness against asymptomatic coronavirus disease 2019 adverse reactions. Additionally, Moderna is in the process of determining safety and efficacy of the Moderna mRNA-1273 COVID-19 vaccine in individuals between the ages of 12 to 18 (*Moderna, Inc, 2021*). In the future, they are also planning clinical studies in pregnant women, individuals under 12 years of age and immunocompromised individuals and all other special risk groups who were excluded from original phase I, II, and III clinical trials (*Moderna, Inc, 2021*).

Chapter 8

Oxford-AstraZeneca Vaccine

Yash Joshi

The Oxford-AstraZeneca vaccine, also called the ChAdOx1 nCoV-19 vaccine (AZD1222), has been under intense scrutiny by various governing bodies around the world. The vaccine was developed at the University of Oxford in partnership with AstraZeneca and is made up of a replication-deficient chimpanzee adenoviral vector (ChAdOx1), which holds the SARS-CoV-2 structural surface glycoprotein antigen, a spike protein gene (nCoV-19) (*Voysey, Clemens, Madhi, Weckx, Zuidewind, et al., 2021*). AstraZeneca is one of the top ten pharmaceutical companies in the world, and it has been extant since 1999 when the merger between Swedish pharmaceutical company, Astra AB, and United Kingdom based Zeneca Group occurred. Production of the vaccine has been dispersed around the world in places such as the United States of America, India, the UK, and various countries in the European Union (*BBC News, 2021a*). It is widely known that the AZD1222 vaccine is less effective than other leading candidates such as the vaccines made by Moderna and Pfizer-BioNTech. The efficacy may be related to how the vaccine works as the Oxford-AstraZeneca vaccine does not rely on mRNA technology like Pfizer-BioNTech and Moderna, rather it uses an adenovirus-vectored technology.

This specific vaccine does have its benefits as well because of its cheap production due to its adenovirus-vectored technology and it can easily be stored in a regular refrigerator. There has been significant hesitancy from numerous people regarding the vaccine produced by Oxford-AstraZeneca due to the adverse effects such as blood clots which have been seen in individuals who have been administered the vaccine.

The Vaccine

This vaccine developed by the University of Oxford and Astra-Zeneca works in a different way than mRNA based vaccines as it is an adenoviral vector-based vaccine. Adenoviruses are viruses that cause non-fatal infections in the epithelium of respiratory, ocular, and gastrointestinal systems in various hosts (*Singh et al., 2018*). These viruses typically only cause mild symptoms in humans, which are why they are usually safe to use (*Dutta, 2021*). These viruses are known to be great vectors for delivering vaccine antigens or genes to a specific tissue. Adenoviruses can be extracted from numerous mammalian species such as chimpanzees and even humans. One of the major benefits associated with adenovirus vaccines is that there is a relatively large and characterized genome available for adenoviruses, meaning that they can easily be genetically modified (*Dutta, 2021*). The Oxford-AstraZeneca vaccine itself is developed from a cold-causing adenovirus which was taken from the stool from chimpanzees (*Callaway, 2020*). When this vaccine gets injected into a human, it instructs cells to produce the SARS-CoV-2 spike protein for COVID-19, which is the immune system's main target (*Callaway, 2020*). Before the adenovirus is injected, it is first modified to ensure that it does not replicate within cells. Overall, the methodology behind the vaccine is based on many successful vaccines that have been developed in the past for other viruses.

Testing of the Vaccine

As with any vaccine, one of the most integral steps are the clinical trials. Clinical trials for the Oxford-AstraZeneca vaccine originally began in the UK, with the UK hosting two trials itself, and then further trials were followed in Brazil and South Africa. The first phase study had an efficacy cohort, while the phase two and three studies also included healthcare workers and other essential workers that had a higher chance of contracting the virus (*Voysey, Clemens, Madhi, Weckx, Zuidewind, et al., 2021*). This approach was used to ensure that trials were being conducted in a safe manner and people were not being put at risk. For the trials ranging from April 23 to November 2020, a total of 23,848 participants were involved cumulatively across all three trial locations (*Voysey, Clemens, Madhi, Weckx, Zuidewind, et al., 2021*). In the secondary UK trial and the Brazil trial, it was seen that most of the participants were aged 18-55, as 86.7% of participants in the UK trial and 89.9% of participants of the Brazil trial, fit that age range (*Voysey, Clemens, Madhi, Weckx, Zuidewind, et al., 2021*). This specific age group was the primary target, as older individuals were targeted in later trials, and there has not been significant data regarding the efficacy of the vaccine on those under the age of 18. Additionally, the participant group consisted of 70.5% female individuals, while 91.4% and 66.6% of those in the UK and Brazil respectively, were white (*Voysey, Clemens, Madhi, Weckx, Zuidewind, et al., 2021*). The lack of diversity amongst the sex of participants as well as race suggests that conclusion from trials regarding the vaccine may not be applicable to all individuals. For example, it would be very difficult to predict adverse effects of the vaccine on a non-Caucasian population, especially since in this situation there is very limited data regarding efficacy within individuals of other races.

Results from Trials

One of the major concerns for hesitancy against the AZD1222 vaccine is related to its efficiency in comparison to the other leading vaccines for COVID-19. Data from clinicals trials for the vaccine showed that after at least one standard dose, 64.1% of participants showed protection against symptomatic disease, with no safety concerns (*Voysey, Clemens, Madhi, Weckx, Zuidewind, et al., 2021*). In general, it was consistently seen that participants who had taken two standard doses in the UK and Brazil had 60.3% and 64.2% efficacy respectively against symptomatic COVID-19 (*Voysey, Clemens, Madhi, Weckx, Zuidewind, et al., 2021*). After the conclusion of more trials, the significant vaccine efficacy of about 70.4% after two doses was seen (*Voysey, Clemens, Madhi, Weckx, Zuidewind, et al., 2021*). In comparison, trials have shown that the Pfizer-BioNTech vaccine has an efficacy of around 85% two weeks after the first dose, while data from patients has shown that the efficiency amount is 89% two weeks after the first dose and then up to 91% 15-28 days after the second dose (*Amit et al., 2021; Petri, 2021*). Similarly, the Moderna vaccine was seen to be 94.1% effective after two doses through its clinical trials (*Oliver et al., 2021*). It is evident that the vaccine prepared by AstraZeneca has been seen to clinically be less effective, which explains some of the hesitancy that many people have towards this specific vaccine.

Blood Clots

Ever since the administration of the Oxford-AstraZeneca vaccine, there have been reports of rare blood clots within individuals. Scientists call the phenomena a vaccine-induced immune thrombotic thrombocytopenia or just thrombosis with thrombocytopenia syndrome (TTS) (*Kupferschmidt & Vogel, 2021*). By March 10, 2021, there were 30 reported cases of thromboembolic events, relating to blood clots, in the five million Oxford-AstraZeneca doses that were administered in Europe (*Wise, 2021*). Some of the earliest cases were reported in women under the age of 60 as most European countries used the shots on educators and healthcare workers, majority who were women (*Kupferschmidt & Vogel, 2021*). In the UK, the frequency of thromboembolic events was greater in those younger than 60, and was reported in about one in every 120,000 Oxford-AstraZeneca vaccine administrations within the country (*Kupferschmidt & Vogel, 2021*). Similar incidence rates were seen in other countries as in Sri Lanka, one in every 150,000 recipients developed the disorder (*Kupferschmidt & Vogel, 2021*). In Germany, there have reports of cerebral venous thrombosis (CVT), which is a stroke related to TTS, in about one in every 76,000 administration of the Oxford-AstraZeneca vaccine. Incidence for CVT was much higher in Norway and Denmark, about one in every 40,000, while there also being an increased chance of other effects related to TTS (*Kupferschmidt & Vogel, 2021*).

There are significant reports and studies which address this connection of blood clots and the Oxford-AstraZeneca vaccine. Data from US health records has shown that the incidence of CVT is greater for those diagnosed with COVID-19 compared to those that receive a vaccine for COVID-19 (*Torjesen, 2021*). In 513,284 patients diagnosed with COVID-19, CVT was seen in 39.0 per million people, while the incidence of CVT in 489,871 individuals who had been administered a COVID-19 vaccine was 4.1 per million (*Taquet et al., 2021*). The vaccines administered to these patients were the Pfizer-BioNTech and Moderna vaccines, and did not include the Oxford-AstraZeneca vaccine. However, the European Medicines Agency has predicted that the incidence of CVT in patients who receive the Oxford-AstraZeneca vaccine would be around 5.0 per million people (*Torjesen, 2021*). It is evident that the risk of blood clots is higher for the Oxford-AstraZeneca vaccine compared to the other mRNA vaccines, yet this risk is substantially lower than developing a blood clot as a result of a COVID-19 diagnosis.

Additionally, there seems to be no clear indication if the risks of blood clots differ between first and second doses of the AstraZeneca vaccine (*Kupferschmidt & Vogel, 2021*). Roughly one in five individuals diagnosed with TTS has died (*Kupferschmidt & Vogel, 2021*). This severe clotting is very difficult to treat outside of a properly equipped hospital, which is why many people in rural areas or with limited healthcare resources will have little support in fighting the condition.

Additionally, a study into the Denmark healthcare system investigated the incidence of venous thromboembolism both before and after the introduction of the Oxford-AstraZeneca vaccine into the population to determine whether or not there was a positive correlation. The study analyzed individuals from January 1, 2010, or their 18th birthday, until their first incident venous thromboembolism, death, emigration, or November 30, 2018, whichever came first (*Østergaard et al., 2021*). These results were compared to the incidence of venous thromboembolism in individuals who received the Oxford-AstraZeneca vaccine up until March 10, 2021 (*Østergaard et al., 2021*). The researchers also calculated incidence rates for venous thromboembolism for all Danish adults, aged 18 years or older censored at the 100th birthday, as well as individuals aged 18–64 years. This specific age group was chosen because it is the age group which has predominantly received the vaccine throughout most European countries, other the UK. The results of this study showed that in a population of 5 million, which is how many people received the Oxford-AstraZeneca vaccine in Europe by March 12, 2021, there would be about 169 expected cases of venous thromboembolism per week, or 736 per month, based in the incidence rate amongst Danish adults aged 18-99 (*Østergaard et al., 2021*). Based on the 18-64 age group, there would be approximately 91 incidents of venous thromboembolism per week , or 398 per month (*Østergaard et al., 2021*). Therefore, although is not possible to completely rule out a relationship between venous thromboembolic events and the Oxford-AstraZeneca vaccine, the data strongly suggests that the number of Europeans who reported thromboembolic events does not seem to have increased due to the usage of the AstraZeneca vaccine. It is believed that the incidence of thromboembolic events would not be significantly lower, at least in the Danish population, without the introduction of the vaccinations.

The Importance of the Vaccine

The prevalence of mRNA vaccines by Pfizer-BioNTech and Moderna had led to questions about the usefulness of the adeno-virus vector based vaccine by AstraZeneca. It is important to note that the Oxford-AstraZeneca vaccine has and will continue to play an important role in ending the pandemic, specifically through the COVAX program. The COVAX program is a global initiative led by the World Health Organization, the Global Vaccine Alliance, and the Coalition for Epidemic Preparedness Innovations (*BBC News, 2021b*). This program was created to make sure that vaccines were distributed equally to both rich and poor nations. The Oxford-AstraZeneca vaccine is expected to make up 50% of the global vaccine supply for lower to middle income nations and a third of the total supply in low-income nations, a big part due to the COVAX program (*Kiernan et al., 2021*). Not only that, a combination of the COVAX program, regional procurement arrangements, and bilateral agreements mean that a total of 180 countries are expected to have access to the Oxford-AstraZeneca vaccine by the end of 2021 (*Kiernan et al., 2021*). Regardless of the concern regarding blood clots, there is still strong global popularity regarding the vaccines. One of the major reasons why is because of the lower price point compared to the likes of other leading vaccine producers such as Moderna and Pfizer-BioNTech. The Oxford-AstraZeneca vaccine costs around $3 to $4 USD a dose, while Pfizer-BioN-Tech and Moderna doses cost anywhere from $15 to $25 USD each (*Irfan, 2020*). Storing the Oxford-AstraZeneca vaccine is also much easier as it can be stored at 2oC to 8oC before puncture (*Ministry of Health, 2021a*). Comparatively, the Pfizer-BioNTech vaccine needs to be stored at -8ooC to -6ooC, while the Moderna vaccine needs to be stored between -25oC and -15oC (*Ministry of Health, 2021b*). From an economic standpoint, the Oxford-AstraZeneca vaccine becomes a more viable option for middle and lower income countries. It also becomes a premier choice for countries that want to quickly inoculate their entire population without spending a luxury amount of money on vaccines like Pfizer-BioNTech and Moderna. For countries in hotter climates, as well as those who cannot accommodate transporting and storing the vaccines at such cold temperatures, the Oxford-AstraZeneca vaccine presents itself as a great opportunity.

Additionally, during the trials of the Oxford-AstraZeneca vaccine, there were certain observations made that would assist the overall vaccination plan for a country. The research team noticed that the results showed no significant difference in efficacy estimates when comparing individuals who had a time interval of less than six weeks between doses, and those who had more than six weeks between doses (*Voysey, Clemens, Madhi, Weckx, Zuidewind, et al., 2021*). The data then suggests that stretching out the interval for vaccine dose administration will not put any lives at risk, and in turn would help countries vaccinate their population more quickly, reducing chances of critical illness and death. Not only that, during the trials it was noticed that an efficacy of 90.0% was seen in individuals who received a lower dose of the Oxford-AstraZeneca vaccine in the UK (*Voysey, Clemens, Madhi, Weckx, Zuidewind, et al., 2021*). A high efficacy for a low dose is very significant because it means that for every vial of vaccine produced, more people can be injected, which can accelerate vaccination programs around the world.

In the UK, the AZD1222 vaccine has been approved for emergency use with two doses given with an interval between 4 and 12 weeks (*Voysey, Clemens, Madhi, Weckx, Group, et al., 2021*). In Canada, the interval between doses is allowed to be extended for up to four months, or about 16 weeks (*Government of Canada, 2021*). Various countries have followed different guidelines in the interval between doses, but there is a possibility that they could follow Canada's lead in extending the interval to up to four months. Data from the phase three efficacy trials in the UK and Brazil, as phase one/two clinical trials in the UK and South Africa up until December 7, 2020 can be used to support their decision. After the first dose of the Oxford-AstraZeneca vaccine, vaccine efficacy was 76% from day 22 to day 90 and it did not seem to change much (*Voysey, Clemens, Madhi, Weckx, Group, et al., 2021*). Antibody levels were also stable during this time period. Additionally, vaccine efficacy was higher in those who were administered standard doses of the vaccine greater than 12 weeks apart compared to those who received the vaccine less than six weeks apart (*Voysey, Clemens, Madhi, Weckx, Group, et al., 2021*). This was supported as more data showed that binding antibody responses were more than 2-fold higher after a period of 12 weeks, compared to less in six weeks in adults aged 18-55 years (*Voysey, Clemens, Madhi, Weckx, Group, et al., 2021*). Overall, these sets of data suggest that extending the interval period between standard doses of the Oxford-AstraZeneca vaccine may be the ideal plan to inoculate the entire population of a country, especially when vaccine supply is limited in many countries.

Future Questions/Developments

The COVID-19 pandemic is a continually evolving situation that may continue to impact many countries worldwide for months or even years to come. There has been an emergence of variants of the virus which have been deadlier and caused more issues in trying to contain the virus. There have been many reports that the current vaccines are not as effective against the emerging variants of the COVID-19 virus. The developers of the Oxford-AstraZeneca vaccine are confident that they will be able to easily modify the vaccine to account for the variants. Chief designer Sarah Gilbert of Oxford University has shared that her team has been working on modifying the vaccine to fight new variants of the virus and they believe that a newer version of the AstraZeneca vaccine will be available in fall 2021 (*D'Agata, 2021*). The reason why the team is so confident that they will be able to make this change is because of the "plug-and-play" platform which is in the original vaccine, where an antigen from a virus for which the vaccine is targeted for, and that is swapped into the original vaccine (*D'Agata, 2021*). These statements seem promising and the vaccine may provide an opportunity for many countries in the near future.

The issues related to blood clots are a concern for the Oxford-AstraZeneca vaccine, and a significant number of countries have acknowledged the issue. Many of the European countries have continually changed their stance on the usage of the Oxford-AstraZeneca vaccine, with numerous countries like France restricting usage to certain age groups. Denmark is the first European country to completely stop the use of the vaccine because of the reports of the rare blood clots (*BBC News, 2021a*). South Africa has stopped its use of the Oxford-AstraZeneca vaccine because of its lack of efficacy against the South African variant (*BBC News, 2021a*). It cannot be said what other countries will follow in stopping the use of the vaccine, or if substantial developments happen such that the vaccine is increasingly used across the world.

Overall, the vaccine created by the University of Oxford and AstraZeneca has played a major role in helping the world fight the pandemic. The use of the adenovirus vector technology makes it a unique vaccine and an effective approach in most scenarios. The vaccine has and will continue to play an integral role in helping the world fight the COVID-19 pandemic, especially in many lower and middle income countries. There will be international attention on this vaccine going forward, specifically if the developers are able to alter it to better combat the variants.

Chapter 9

Sputnik: Out With the Space Satellite, in With the Vaccine

Marcey Costello

THE SPUTNIK COVID-19 vaccine, uncommonly known as the Gam-COVID-Vac (*Jones & Roy, 2021, p. 642*), is one of many vaccines circulating the world, but it is the only one developed in Russia. "The vaccine is named after the first Soviet space satellite. The launch of Sputnik-1 in 1957 reinvigorated space research around the world" (*The Gamaleya Center, n.d.*). The Gamaleya National Research Center for Epidemiology and Microbiology (*Gamaleya NRCEM*) in Moscow, Russia created the two-dose vaccine to be administered twenty-one days apart and is available "in more than [sixty] countries" (*Jones & Roy, 2021, p. 642; The Gamaleya Center, n.d.*). The *Gamaleya NRCEM*, founded in 1891, is one of the world's leading research institutions (*The Gamaleya Center, n.d.*). The increasing numbers of COVID-19 cases worldwide have caused countries to push for vaccine approval including Russia, Belarus, and Argentina where "Sputnik V received regulatory approval" (*Rogliani, Chetta, Cazzola, & Calzetta, 2021, p. 228*). According to Jones and Roy, the Sputnik vaccine is different from other common vaccines because it uses two varying serotypes rather than the same material for both doses (*2021, p. 642*). Logunov explains that "the use of two immunisations gives a durable and long-lasting immune response" (2021, 672). Sputnik uses adenovirus twenty-six (Ad26) and adenovirus five (Ad5) as vectors in its doses which, simply, means modified DNA from viruses found in adenoid tissue (i.e. the lining of eyes, airways, and lungs) to make the vaccine effective without the recipient contracting COVID-19 (*Jones & Roy, 2021, p. 642; Oxford University Press, 2021; Shroff, 2020; Centers for Disease Control and Prevention, 2021*). The vaccine is injected into the shoulder muscle like other vaccines, normally referred to as intramuscular injection, for the quickest absorption into the body (*Logunov, 2021, pp. 672-673*).

To determine the efficacy of the Sputnik vaccine, a trial was conducted with three phases (*Logunov, 2021, p. 672*). The first phase started on June seventeenth, 2020, and was completed on August tenth, 2020 (*Gamaleya Research Institute of Epidemiology and Microbiology, 2020*). The first phase was non-randomized and only consisted of thirty-eight participants (*Gamaleya Research Institute of Epidemiology and Microbiology, 2020*). The first stage of phase one included nine volunteers who received the first dose of the Sputnik vaccine (*Gamaleya Research Institute of Epidemiology and Microbiology, 2020*). The second group also consisted of nine volunteers who received the second dose of the Sputnik vaccine (*Gamaleya Research Institute of Epidemiology and Microbiology, 2020*). The vaccines were administered in a hospital in Moscow, Russia and the volunteers were monitored for the following five days to ensure the safety of the vaccine (*Gamaleya Research Institute of Epidemiology and Microbiology, 2020*). "Based on the results of the safety assessment, the Chief investigator [decided] to proceed to the second stage of the study on the 5th day after the introduction of the studied drugs" (*Gamaleya Research Institute of Epidemiology and Microbiology, 2020*). The second stage of phase one included the remaining twenty volunteers who were vaccinated five days after the two groups from stage one

(*Gamaleya Research Institute of Epidemiology and Microbiology, 2020*). The twenty volunteers received the first dose of the Sputnik vaccine and, twenty-one days later, received the second dose (*Gamaleya Research Institute of Epidemiology and Microbiology, 2020*). They were required to complete four follow-up visits "7, 14, 28, [and] 42 days after administration of the drug" to ensure its efficacy and safety (*Gamaleya Research Institute of Epidemiology and Microbiology, 2020*).

The third phase of the trials started on September seventh, 2020 (*Logunov, 2021, p. 676*). To find participants, the Moscow Government used an online platform along with community outreach efforts and call centers (*Logunov, 2021, p. 672*). The trial used randomly selected participants along with a placebo to be administered to some participants (i.e. the participant believed they were receiving the Sputnik vaccine when it was actually an inactive solution) (*Logunov, 2021, p. 672*). The third phase was conducted at twenty-five hospitals and polyclinics (i.e. centers providing primary and secondary healthcare) in Moscow, Russia which were approved by the Ministry of Health of the Russian Federation (*Logunov, 2021, p. 672*; *Oxford University Press, 2021*). Twenty-one-thousand nine-hundred and seventy-seven participants met the extensive eligibility criteria, were screened, and signed explicit consent forms before the phase began (*Logunov, 2021, pp. 673-674*). The eligibility criteria included being eighteen years or older, negative test results of HIV, hepatitis C and B, syphilis, COVID-19, pregnancy, alcohol, and drugs along with not having been in contact with a person diagnosed with COVID-19 within the last fourteen days and no history of COVID-19 (*Logunov, 2021, p. 673*). The exclusion criteria included receiving any vaccination or steroids in the thirty days prior to enrolment, pregnancy or breastfeeding, tuberculosis, or an allergy to the drug itself or its components (*Logunov, 2021, p. 673*). The exclusion and eligibility criteria were extensive to ensure the health and safety of the volunteers and the accuracy of the results (i.e. the results were not impeded by participants with COVID-19); the criterion were the same for phases one and two of the trials (*Gamaleya Research Institute of Epidemiology and Microbiology, 2020*). To ensure the groups of participants were randomized effectively, the participants were first divided into age categories of eighteen to thirty years old, thirty-one to forty-years-old, forty-one to fifty-years-old, fifty-one to sixty-years old, and sixty-years old and above (*Logunov, 2021, p. 673*). They were then assigned randomly generated identification numbers by a computer program (*Logunov, 2021, p. 673*). Finally, the vaccine and placebo were in identical packaging to ensure the participants and administrators were unaware of who was receiving what (*Logunov, 2021, p. 673*). The phase lasted for one-hundred and eighty days where the participants were required to complete one screening visit (i.e. physical examination, blood test, urine sample, etc. - to keep a health record) and five on-site visits to a designated clinic (*Logunov, 2021, p. 673*). During the on-site visits, the participants' vital signs were taken and general questions regarding their wellbeing were posed (*Logunov, 2021, p. 673*). They experienced the same procedure when they received the second dose twenty-one days after the first (*Logunov, 2021, p. 673*). If the participant tested positive for COVID-19, they were ineligible to receive the second dose and were seen by medical staff for treatment (*Logunov, 2021, p. 673*). The only times the participants were tested for COVID-19 was at the beginning of the trial, at the twenty-one-day mark, and if they were symptomatic (*Logunov, 2021, p. 673*). The participants were able to contact telemedicine staff (i.e. trial staff who communicate electronically) to ask questions or voice concerns about the trial procedures at any point during the one-hundred and eighty days (*Logunov, 2021, p. 673; Oxford University Press, 2021*). Participants were also given instructions on how to download an application on their smartphone that helped them monitor their own wellbeing (*Logunov, 2021, p. 674*). Those who did not use the application were contacted by the trial staff on a regular basis (*Logunov, 2021, p. 674*). The city of

Moscow uses an electronic health record (EHR) which acts as a medical record of Moscow's citizens used by the healthcare providers in the city (*Logunov, 2021, p. 674*). The trial staff updated the EHRs of the participants to indicate their participation and to track their wellbeing in case they required an ambulance or visited a healthcare provider outside of their scheduled visits (*Logunov, 2021, p. 674*). The trial staff included the participants' smartphone monitoring application in their EHRs to further ensure and monitor the participants' health (*Logunov, 2021, p. 674*).

Out of the twenty-one-thousand nine-hundred and seventy-seven participants, five-thousand four-hundred and seventy-six received the placebo and sixteen-thousand five-hundred and one received the Sputnik vaccine (*Logunov, 2021, p. 676*). On November eighth, 2020, twenty cases of COVID-19 were reported (*Logunov, 2021, p. 676*). On November twenty-fourth, 2020, seventy-eight cases of COVID-19 were reported (*Logunov, 2021, p. 676*). On day twenty-one of the trial when participants were given the second dose, there were sixteen confirmed COVID-19 cases in the group that received Sputnik and sixty-two confirmed cases in the group that received the placebo (*Logunov, 2021, p. 676*). By day twenty-one, the Sputnik vaccine had an efficacy rate of 91.6% (*Logunov, 2021, p. 676*). "Notably, in the vaccine group, most cases of COVID-19 occurred before dose [two]" (*Logunov, 2021, p. 677*). "The most common [side effects of the vaccine] were flu-like illness, injection site reactions, headache, and asthenia" (i.e. lack of strength and energy) after the second dose (*Logunov, 2021, p. 678; Oxford University Press, 2021*). Throughout the study, there were four deaths in total with three being in the vaccine group and one being in the placebo group, but Logunov assures, "No vaccine-related deaths were reported" (*2021, p. 678*). The Gamaleya NRCEM reports that there were "[n]o serious adverse events associated with the vaccination, as confirmed by [the] Independent Data Monitoring Committee" and that there were "[n]o strong allergies" nor "anaphylactic shock" (n.d.). Jones and Roy conclude that *"[t]he trial results show [a] consistent strong protective effect across all participant age groups" (Jones & Roy, 2021, p. 642).*

One of the main concerns individuals have with the Sputnik vaccine is the way in which it was developed: Russia did not consult The World Health Organization (WHO), the European Medicines Agency (EMA), or any other organization interested in vaccination development and approval (*Balakrishnan, 2020, p. 1128; Holt, 2021, p. 958*). Organizations such as WHO and EMA help determine the risks and efficacy of the vaccines while also implementing health policies and evaluating applications for potentially marketable products (*European Medicines Agency, n.d.; World Health Organization, n.d.*). Logunov explains that "the vaccine candidate was provisionally approved in Russia according to national legislation" along with being approved by the Department of State Regulation for Circulation of Medicines of the Ministry of Health of the Russian Federation, the Moscow City Independent Ethics Committee, and other clinics and ethics committees (*2021, p. 672*). But without the consultation of credible organizations like WHO and EMA, there is no guarantee that policies and regulations were followed and the vaccine is safe for humans. Thomas Cunei, a member of the International Federation of Pharmaceutical Manufacturers and Associations in Geneva, Switzerland, states, "no matter how urgently action is needed against the COVID-19 public health emergency, it is imperative for the vaccine makers to [uphold] the highest standards of quality, safety, and efficacy" (*Balakrishnan, 2020, p. 1128*). Cunei also expresses that the "[l]ack of transparency on results of preclinical or clinical trials, let alone transparency on due process remains concerning" (B*alakrishnan, 2020, p. 1128*). Additionally, the chairman of Slovakia's Doctors Trade Union, Peter Visolajsky, states, *"If a patient came to me and asked about the Sputnik vaccine, I would say that I could not recommend it because it hasn't been through an approval process. It may be a good and effective vaccine, but it's not registered, so we don't have* data...for it'" (*Holt, 2021, p. 958*). A citizen of Bratislava, Slovakia voiced their concerns to The Lancet as well, "*'Other vaccines have gone through a process of approval with the EMA, but Sputnik V has not. I don't trust the quality of the vaccine itself, nor the conditions under which the doses might be produced, stored, or transported'*" (*Holt, 2021, p. 958*). A virologist at the Czech Academy of Sciences, Libor Grubhoffer, also voiced similar concerns to The Lancet, "'It should not be used until a proper approval procedure has taken place, for example by the EMA'" (*Holt, 2021, p.958*). People are unwilling to receive Sputnik unless it undergoes the same approval process that the other COVID-19 vaccines have gone through; whether it be approved by WHO or EMA does not matter as long as it is a credible organization.

Another concern that individuals have regarding Russia's vaccine is the contradictory results. In other words, many articles have been written regarding Russia's vaccine, but they all contradict each other because some express the vaccine's efficacy while others say that it is not effective. On one hand, Balakrishnan explains that "S*putnik V's safety in rhesus macaque monkeys, rabbits, guinea pigs, rats, and mice, and its efficacy in marmoset monkeys and Gamaleya's own immune-suppressed Syrian golden hamsters, [observed] a 100% protection from a high degree of infection*" (*2020, p. 1128*). A thorough analysis conducted on the phase three trials of the vaccine concluded with a "*91·6% efficacy against COVID-19 and [that it] was well tolerated in a large cohort*" (**Logunov, 2021, p. 671**). Logunov states, "*Our results also showed that the vaccine was 100%...efficacious against severe COVID-19, although this was a secondary outcome as the results are preliminary*" (*2021, p. 679*). "*[T]he developers [even] claim [Sputnik] to be the 'best vaccine' against COVID-19*" (*Balakrishnan, 2020, p. 1128*). The Gamaleya National Research Center for Epidemiology and Microbiology affirms, "*Sputnik V is one of the three vaccines in the world with efficacy over 90%*" (n.d.). On the other hand, Balakrishnan states, "*Sheena Cruickshank, an immunologist at University of Manchester, UK, thinks* *that the results of this open-labelled, non-randomised study over-estimate treatment effects of Sputnik V"* and that *"the variable and insignificant levels of neutralising antibodies are concerning"* (*2020, p. 1128*). The fact that scientists cannot come to an agreement on the efficacy of Sputnik concerns the potential recipients of the vaccine.

Moreover, there is concern that the Sputnik vaccine will not be effective in thwarting the COVID-19 variants. One article explains that *"Benhur Lee at the Icahn School of Medicine at Mount Sinai in New York City and his colleagues obtained samples of anti-body-laden blood serum from 12 people vaccinated with Sputnik V"* (*Nature, 2021*). Lee's team concluded that the vaccine did not impede the South African variant B.1.351 but that it neutralized the British variant B.1.1.7 (*Nature, 2021*). Therefore, scientists are unable to come to a conclusion about whether Sputnik is an effective vaccine or not which is a grave concern for those who will receive the vaccine. The lack of clarity causes people to wonder what the next step will be after they receive the vaccine if it only helps with COVID-19 and one of the variants. In other words, protection against the variants of COVID-19 is becoming just as important as protection against the original virus because the variants are becoming more common across the globe as of *"the end of 2020"* (*Moore, 2021, p. 1251*). While Sputnik *"induced a very large effect on the level of neutralizing antibodies"* against COVID-19, it cannot be *"quickly re-engineered to mimic new mutations"* like the Oxford-AstraZeneca, Pfizer, and Moderna vaccines can (*Rogliani, Chetta, Cazzola, & Calzetta, 2021, p. 227*). Potential recipients of Sputnik want to know that the vaccine will protect them and that if it cannot, it can be re-engineered to.

The uncertainty surrounding the lack of consultation with credible organizations like WHO and EMA leads people to wonder if the vaccine is safe for humans. Will WHO or EMA be conducting their own analyses of the vaccine? Will they be monitoring further Sputnik trials? When will the public know if Sputnik meets the approval of WHO, EMA, and other credible organizations? Were proper safety regulations and policies implemented in the development of Sputnik to the approval of WHO and EMA? Receiving a vaccine is integral to ending the pandemic, but if the vaccine is unsafe should people be receiving it?

As previously mentioned, the Oxford-AstraZeneca, Pfizer, and Moderna vaccines can be "quickly re-engineered to mimic new mutations" but the Sputnik vaccine cannot be (*Rogliani, Chetta, Cazzola, & Calzetta, 2021, p. 227*). Its lack of efficacy toward other COVID-19 variants concerns the potential recipients of the vaccine because it is not completely reliable nor easily modified for further variant-specific doses. One unanswered question is: Will the Sputnik vaccine developers create a new formula to overcome the other COVID-19 variants? If they do, will it go through WHO and EMA's approval process? Furthermore, will further studies be conducted to determine more concrete evidence on the efficacy of Sputnik?

Additionally, despite knowing some of the short-term side effects of the vaccines, what will the long-term side effects be and when will they be made known? Will it be months or years before recipients know the long-term effects? Will research be conducted to determine the long-term side effects? Moreover, can research be conducted to determine the long-term side effects?

There are many unanswered questions concerning the Sputnik COVID-19 vaccine and much uncertainty about the direction its future will take. Will it continue to be purchased by other countries to inoculate their citizens? Will it undergo further testing and trials? Will there be more thorough analyses of trials that will then be published and made available to the public? Will Russian citizens be able to receive a different COVID-19 vaccine as opposed to Sputnik?

The Sputnik vaccine, developed in Moscow, Russia by the Gamaleya National Research Center for Epidemiology and Microbiology, is one of the many COVID-19 vaccines quickly developed to combat the illness (*Jones & Roy, 2021, p. 642*). The lack of WHO or EMA approval coupled with the contradictory results concerning Sputnik's efficacy rates and its inability to be re-engineered quickly to account for the variants raise concerns for potential recipients (*Rogliani, Chetta, Cazzola, & Calzetta, 2021, p. 227*). Without WHO or EMA approval, potential recipients of Sputnik worry about their safety. In addition, Sputnik's inability to be quickly re-engineered like the Oxford-AstraZeneca, Pfizer, and Moderna vaccines causes people to wonder if the vaccine should be used at all (*Rogliani, Chetta, Cazzola, & Calzetta, 2021, p. 227*). There are questions that need to be answered and not enough people to answer them. Potential vaccine recipients need clear answers with evidence to support those answers in order to be confident that the vaccine they will receive is safe for them and that it will combat COVID-19. Without such reassurances, there is little doubt that people will not want to receive the Sputnik vaccine even if it may be their only option depending on where they live.

Chapter 10

Vaccine Hesitancy

Armita Yousefi

A FTER EXAMINING DIFFERENT vaccines in the previous chapters, it is essential to investigate the factors that could impact the administration of vaccines. In 2019, the World Health Organization (WHO) declared vaccine hesitancy to be one of the ten threats to global health. Vaccine hesitancy refers to "the delay in acceptance or refusal of vaccines despite availability of vaccine services" (*Macdonald & SAGE working group, 2015*). As shown in Figure 1, the continuum of vaccine hesitancy is essential to distinguish. Vaccine hesitancy rarely refers to the refusal of all vaccines and merely encompasses the following criteria: accept some not all, delay, and refuse some not all (*Macdonald & SAGE working group, 2015*). The factors that impact vaccine hesitancy are very much dependent on the representation of vaccines. The government officials and social media dictate this representation, especially with the inevitable growth of globalization. It is important to preface this discussion by stating that vaccine hesitancy manifests in various conditions worldwide, and location is an essential factor to consider. Location is critical in terms of the resources available to provide vaccines, and there are cultural differences that contribute to the hesitancy for vaccination.

High Demand   No Demand

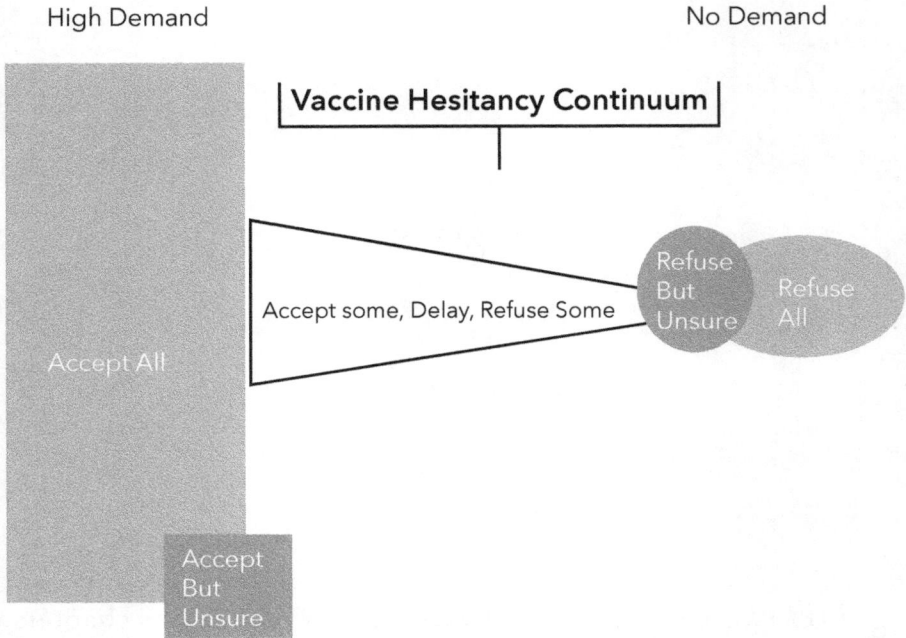

FIGURE 1: *The continuum of vaccine hesitancy between full acceptance and outright refusal of all vaccines*
Note. From MacDonald, N. E., & the SAGE Working Group on Vaccine Hesitancy (2015) [The continuum of vaccine hesitancy between full acceptance and outright refusal of all vaccines]. Vaccine.
https://doi.org/10.1016/j.vaccine.2015.04.036

The root of vaccine hesitancy is based on the information and data available to the public through research papers. Therefore, the discussion of this topic will not include misinformation rather the analysis of the information that is provided by the government and the research done by the vaccination companies. There are many valid concerns surrounding the COVID-19 vaccinations that are in the process of being administered due to the examination of the internal validity and external validity of the research for these vaccines. Nevertheless, vaccine hesitancy will damage the desired outcomes of the vaccination process in immunizing the population. As discussed in previous chapters, the importance of vaccination during the COVID-19 pandemic is both for personal protection and the protection of others. Vaccine hesitancy would be a challenge to achieving herd immunity. The more vulnerable demographics that are most prone to experience the harsh results of the virus can only be fully immunized if others around them are immunized against the virus as well.

The SAGE working group has presented the three main factors that impact vaccine hesitancy: complacency, convenience, and confidence (2014). These three factors are the main determinants of vaccine hesitancy, and each factor has many subcategories (*Macdonald & SAGE working group, 2015*). The following diagram exhibits the "3Cs" model of vaccine hesitancy's determinants and reveals the multilayered impact of the three factors.

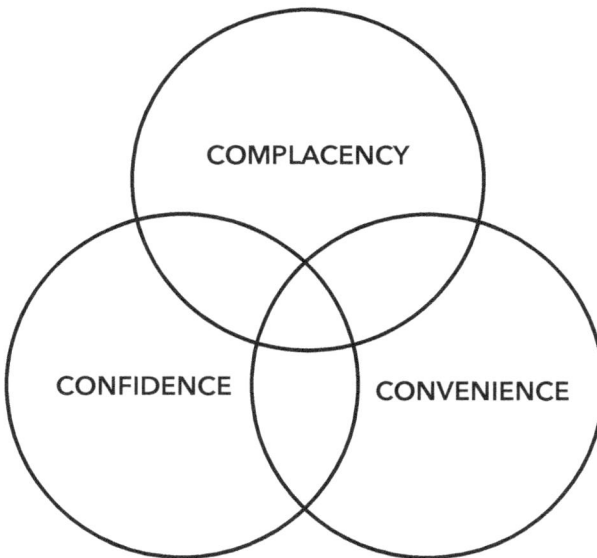

FIGURE 2: *"Three Cs" model of vaccine hesitancy*
Note. From MacDonald, N. E., & the SAGE Working Group on Vaccine Hesitancy (2015) ["Three Cs" model of vaccine hesitancy]. Vaccine.
https://doi.org/10.1016/j.vaccine.2015.04.036

Complacency affects vaccine hesitancy when individuals believe that the vaccination of the virus does not successfully prevent the spread of the virus and the anticipated risks of the virus are low (*Macdonald & SAGE working group, 2015*). In the case of COVID-19 vaccination, vaccine complacency is mainly impacted by misinformation, such as individuals who are against wearing masks in public areas. Much of this information leads to conspiracy theories which will be discussed in the following chapter. However, there are cases of complacency in which misinformation is not the leading cause. An important example of this is the slow vaccine roll-out rate for New Zealand that has allowed vaccination for less than 4% of their population despite their successful approach to preventing large outbreaks during the pandemic (Hollingsworth, 2021). This percentage is extremely low, especially compared to other regions that suffered significantly from the impacts of the COVID-19 pandemic. For example, the United Kingdom has vaccinated 47% of its population despite the many cases and deaths it has suffered in the past year (Hollingsworth, 2021). There are many reasons for the low rate of vaccinations in New Zealand. One of them is the availability of the vaccines, as New Zealand did not rush to purchase vaccines due to the low numbers of cases and deaths (Hollingsworth, 2021). The leaders believe that they benefit from waiting to vaccinate their population to observe the impact that it could have (Hollingsworth, 2021). New Zealand can afford the delayed vaccination roll-out as the pandemic conditions are not impacting them compared to other regions; this effectively falls under vaccine complacency.

Another example of vaccine complacency that contributes to hesitancy and is not the result of misinformation is the concept of self-efficacy. Self-efficacy describes the ability of an individual to take action on behalf of themselves to be vaccinated (*Macdonald & SAGE working group, 2015*). This definition is not strictly under vaccine complacency and overlaps with the convenience factor of vaccine hesitancy. However, there is a distinction to be made in which vaccine convenience targets a large population, whereas self-efficacy is the perceived or actual ability of an individual. An example of this would be an individual who is confused about booking an appointment for their vaccination due to the unclear instructions provided by the health care service. As a result, this individual might be less inclined to book their appointment or delay the process due to the confusion caused by the process.

The ability to access vaccination for a population rather than an individual as mentioned previously belongs to the category of vaccine convenience. The inability to obtain vaccination whether it is limited in terms of geographical distance, affordability, and vaccine and service availability (*Macdonald & SAGE working group, 2015*). These factors are very much dependent on the regional services provided by the government and differ from country to country. In more developed countries, accessibility to the vaccine is much higher, and therefore many are more inclined to get vaccinated. A study showed that the lowest acceptance rate for the COVID-19 vaccines was in the Middle East, Russia, Africa, and some countries in Europe (*Sallam, 2021*). The lowest acceptance rate was reported in the Middle East; Kuwait obtains 23.6% vaccine acceptance (*Sallam, 2021*). Although the study did not indicate a reason for this low rate, a reason could stem from the availability of vaccines. It is important to note that this is not the sole reason for this low vaccine acceptance rate and there are other factors such as mistrust in the government in the Middle East (*Schaer, 2021*). Recently, the second shipment of the Pfizer vaccine for Kuwait was delayed and around 27% of the population has received at least one dose of the vaccine (*Schaer, 2021*). This would entail that around 13% of the population has been fully vaccinated with 1 million doses administered and a total population of 4 million (*Schaer, 2021*). Thus, the low vaccine availability could explain the low vaccine acceptance rate in Kuwait.

Vaccine confidence is the most significant factor that impacts vaccine hesitancy in the age of COVID-19. There are three ways in which confidence can be manifested in vaccine hesitancy: confidence in the vaccines, confidence in the medical professionals who administer the vaccines, and confidence in the scientists who develop and study the vaccines (*Smith, 2017*). It is essential to note that in the case of COVID-19 the confidence in the vaccines and the confidence in the scientists who develop and study the vaccines overlap as the research available to the public is the only source of information for the recently developed vaccines.

Concerns of confidence in the medical professionals who administer the vaccines can be attributed to the increasing mistrust in the medical system with the increasing access to education and the internet (*Sweeney, 2018*). In 2012, 34% of Americans trusted their leaders in the medical field which is a significant drop from the 73% of Americans who trusted their leaders in 1996 (*Blenden et al., 2014*). This shocking statistic reveals that with the increase of technological advances, there has been more information about the failure of this institution along with others, mainly concerning the self-interest of the health care system, the insurers, and professional organizations, namely the American Medical Association (*Sweeney, 2018*). Furthermore, with a higher rate of accessibility to the internet, the general public is more likely to question their health care professional as they can access many websites that identify diagnosis and course of treatment (*Sweeney, 2018*). However, this does allow for misinformation to influence the general public and therefore this lack of trust may be a result of misinformation from the internet.

An example specific to COVID-19 vaccines that could have resulted in further distrust in the medical practitioners who administer the vaccines occurred in Ontario. The Mackenzie Health hospital broadcasted a message that on March 28th, six people who were to be vaccinated were accidentally injected with saline solution (*Pope, 2021*). Although the saline solution is harmless to the body and those who were impacted by this did receive their vaccination later, this could have decreased the initial confidence that many in the Mackenzie Health administrators. Due to the delayed shipment of Pfizer vaccines in January, the vaccination plan for Ontario was hampered and resulted in further delays (*Office of the Premier, 2021*). Since the Mackenzie Health hospital has been one of the main administrators of vaccines, the lack of confidence from the general population in the ability of this center further caused the hampering of the vaccination plan that the Ontario Government has proposed.

Another main concern surrounding the confidence in medical practitioners can be loosely applied to confidence in the research of the vaccine as well. An example that encompasses this questioning of confidence came about when Canada's COVID-19 vaccine task force revealed its conflict of interest (*Lexchin et al., 2020*). Many questioned whether those with a conflict of interest should be on the task force as the decisions made by those officials in choosing the vaccines will influence the entire population; therefore it can be argued that this decision should not be influenced by the conflict of interest held by the members. This can both impact the confidence that the population has in the task force and also the chosen vaccines to be administered as they could be influenced by the conflict of interest present (*Lexchin et al., 2020*).

The confidence in the researchers of the vaccine can be influenced by the extent of the internal and external validities of the studies. Whereas internal validity assesses the success of a study to establish a cause and effect relationship, external validity measured the generalizability of the research (*Cuncic, 2020*). The internal validity of a research paper is dependent on whether the study has been successful in establishing a cause and effect relationship between the two variables and in the case of vaccine research, the conflict of interest present in research papers and in the medical practitioners who endorse the vaccines as previously mentioned could impact the internal validity. However, in the case of the COVID-19 vaccines presented, the internal validity is not impacted severely and there is a high internal validity observed in the vaccine research.

The main concern surrounding the COVID-19 vaccine research is external validity. External validity examines how effectively the research can show successful results as it did in the research. One of the most recent concerns with the external validity of the research is how well can the vaccines adapt to the new mutations and variants of the SARS-CoV-2 virus (*Hewings-Martin & Cohut, 2021*). There have been many variants that have been emerging around the world, the most notable one being the B.1.1.7 variant emerging from The United Kingdom (*Hewings-Martin & Cohut, 2021*). Although researchers cannot identify the process or the specific efficacy rate of the protection of the BNT162b2 mRNA vaccine (Pfizer vaccine) against the variant, they have identified that there is a certain degree of effectiveness (*Dagan et al., 2021*). Although this research paper has made this discovery about the effectiveness of one of the vaccines on the new variant, there have been many more mutations causing the number of variants to increase worldwide. These include variants such as the B.1.617, first identified in India, and B.1.351, originating from South Africa (*Hewings-Martin & Cohut, 2021*). The efficacy of the vaccine against the other variants, specifically B.1.351, proves to be much lower than against the B.1.1.7 variant. A study shows that the Oxford-AstraZeneca only had 10.1% efficacy against this strain; however, it is important to note that this study does not show high internal validity due to the small sample size and the lack of the peer-reviewing process (*Hewings-Martin & Cohut, 2021*). This could be a source of questioning the vaccines and their efficacy against the new developing strains as there seems to be a constant state of mutation that causes the variants to emerge. A future direction that has already taken place with determining how the vaccines can adapt to the new variants is the development of new vaccines to observe their effectiveness against the B.1.351. Moderna is in the process of researching and testing their new developmental vaccine against this variant as it is relatively not difficult to modify mRNA vaccines to increase efficacy against the new variants (*Hewings-Martin & Cohut, 2021*). Although this step is a very important step towards tackling this issue, there is a concern with how these vaccines could be administered if proved to be successful and what the guideline would be for these newly modified vaccines. Therefore, many could be hesitant to get vaccinated due to the low efficacy shown towards the new strains of the SARS-CoV-2 virus depending on their place of residence and the development of the variants in their country.

Another concern surrounding the research of the COVID-19 vaccines that could impact vaccine hesitancy significantly is the representation of demographics in the research. The BNT162b2 vaccine (Pfizer-BioNTech) provided the demographic of their participants based on their sex, race, country, age, and body-mass index (*Polack et al., 2020*). The percentage of female and male participants was very close, 48.9% and 51.1% respectively (*Polack et al., 2020*). The lack of inclusion of the intersex population could deter some of the population from receiving the vaccine as this demographic has not been tested on. Furthermore, the female population excluded pregnant people and this would contribute to the hesitancy for pregnant females to obtain the vaccine due to its lack of testing on their demographic (*Polack et al., 2020*). Additionally, the lack of immunocompromised persons in the research further prevents that demographic to gain confidence in the vaccine (*Polack et al., 2020*). The lack of long-term research for the COVID-19 vaccines is also another significant enabler of vaccine hesitancy. The safety and efficacy of the BNT162b2 vaccine were only tested for 2 months in the trials of the vaccine and therefore the longer-term impact of the vaccine could not be identified (*Polack et al., 2020*). Another concern is the transmission of the virus. Although the vaccine offers protection against symptomatic COVID-19, the protection against asymptomatic infection is unknown and untested and this would create a big concern for those who are skeptical about the vaccine (*Polack et al., 2020*). Thus the external validity of the research done for the vaccines is questionable due to the limited time and has created lots of hesitancy towards the efficacy of the vaccines.

There are many valid reasons for people to delay their vaccination, and deny or accept only some vaccines as the research for the vaccines have been conducted in a short period of time. To reiterate, the three factors impacting vaccine hesitancy are complacency, convenience, and confidence. The three factors are not isolated, and in many cases, there is a combination of these factors that truly impact the opinions of people on their choice to get vaccinated. These concerns do not originate from misinformation yet from the limited scope of research done on the COVID-19 vaccines. Perhaps with research that includes a larger demographic and longer trials, there would be more assurance of how well the vaccines can adapt. Therefore, there could be a possibility of reducing the impact of vaccine hesitancy with the right action taken from researchers, medical practitioners, and government officials. In the next chapter, the spread of conspiracy theories that arise from misinformation about the COVID-19 vaccines will be examined.

Chapter 11

Conspiracy Theories surrounding COVID-19 vaccines

Dasarathy Mutharasan

THE EFFECTIVENESS OF vaccines has been documented over several centuries, with the first vaccines having been developed in the early 90s (*The Children's Hospital of Philadelphia, 2014*). They have enabled the extinction of various diseases like polio and smallpox. However, skepticism and conspiracy theories have encumbered vaccination efforts. These conspiracy theories often manipulate some elements of the truth to cater to the fears and mistrust of niche demographics. Furthermore, the theories utilize fear-mongering and exaggerated headlines to grab the attention of people. All of these factors lead to the viral spread of these conspiracy theories that are often based on no real evidence. This chapter will break down various conspiracies that surround the COVID-19 vaccines, the factors that lead to the spread of these theories. Later, potential solutions will be explored to address this misinformation epidemic.

Amplification of Conspiracy Theories on Social Media and Internet

The internet and social media have vastly extended the reach of vaccination campaigns. The public can access information regarding COVID-19, public health measures, and more with a few clicks. However, the democratization of information has also amplified anti-vaccine attitudes globally. Clickbait articles and sensationalized titles can spread with the help of online algorithms that push anti-vaccine content to individuals that are receptive to this type of content. A paper by Burki (*2020*) reported that "*31 million people follow anti-vaccine groups on Facebook*" while 17 million people subscribe to similar content on Youtube. Interestingly enough, some research suggests that only a small number of individuals are responsible for a large majority of the anti-vaccine campaigns that circulate online. According to a report by the CCDH (*2021*), an analysis of over 800,000 posts from Facebook and Twitter found that only 12 individuals are responsible for 65% of anti-vaccine content. These are high-profile individuals with millions on top of millions of followers—for instance, influencer and dietary supplement entrepreneur Joseph Mercola has a combined following of 3.6 million people.

The Immune Booster Craze

A recurring conspiracy theory that has populated social media and the internet is that vitamins and dietary supplements like zinc are viable cures that can replace public health measures and vaccines. This has grown especially popular, as demand has increased for "immune-boosters" or foods that promote a strong immune system. This has led to a conflict between commercial purposes and staying true to health science. The FDA (*2021*) put out a public warning letter to Joseph Mercola to stop marketing supplements like "Liposomal Vitamin C" and Vitamin D supplements as a treatment of COVID-19. Mercola has a net worth of $100 million and is only one of many influencers that have leveraged their following to rake in millions of dollars in profits. He donated $2.9 million to the oldest anti-vaccine organization, National Vaccine Information Centre, and $4 million to several other organizations that spread similar anti-vaccine sentiment (*Sun & Satija, 2019*). While the exact dollar of this anti-vaccine industry is unknown, the industry is incredibly lucrative. The methods that influencers use to make a living are numerous, from pills to supplements to books to seminars and more. The leveraging of people's mistrust and fears to generate profits is quite insidious especially when the theories and information that is spread are completely baseless. Rather than promoting balanced conversations that take into account many perspectives, an echo chamber is quickly developed. Anti-vaccine headlines and studies are cherry-picked to match an agenda that sows mistrust in public health authorities and current health guidelines. Consequently, influencers can market various goods from supplements that promise immunity to an amazing book that explains how the pandemic is a hoax. When taking a closer look at these theories that have circulated, they quickly break down. For instance, many influencers claim that alternative medicines can be used to protect against COVID-19 like zinc or vitamin D. In reality, there has been no conclusive evidence regarding the relationship between vitamin D and COVID-19, as various studies have come to different conclusions (*Rubin 2021*). Research studies in France and Spain that examined 77 patients with COVID-19 found that vitamin D supplements were correlated with better survival. In another case, a study in Italy found that there was no association between vitamin D and COVID-19. Surprisingly, one study correlated a greater health risk to vitamin D supplements.

It is important to note that a balanced diet containing all of the essential vitamins and minerals will help maximize an individual's immune system (*Childs et al., 2019*)—for instance, zinc assists in the cell division of antibodies that make up our immune system. However, the conspiracy theory that consuming vitamin and mineral supplements can replace public health measures and vaccinations is not backed by scientific research. A healthy person, fortified by supplements, can still contract the virus. Even if they survive it, they can still spread it to other immunocompromised individuals. The effects of this theory can be devastating as individuals are inclined to spread conspiracy theories to other individuals and ignore public health mandates to continue spreading the virus.

The Conspiracy of 5G microchips hidden in vaccines

Another theory that has circulated the internet is that vaccines are a ploy by billionaire Bill Gates to inject people with 5G microchips, unknownst to them (*Goodman & Flora, 2020*).

December 27,2020

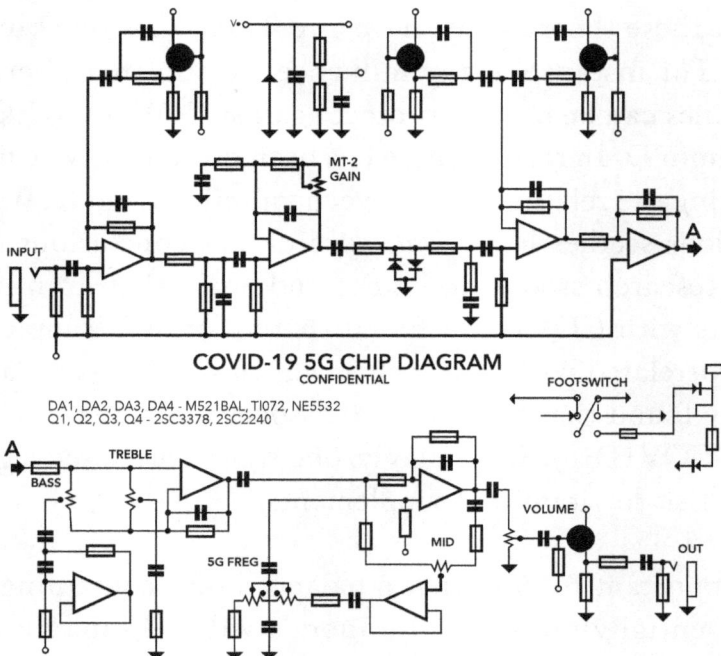

COVID-19 5G CHIP DIAGRAM
CONFIDENTIAL

FIGURE 1: *This diagram, supposedly portraying the 5G chip embedded in the vaccine, went viral in various countries. However, it was debunked that this was the circuit board of a guitar pedal (**Smith, 2021**).*

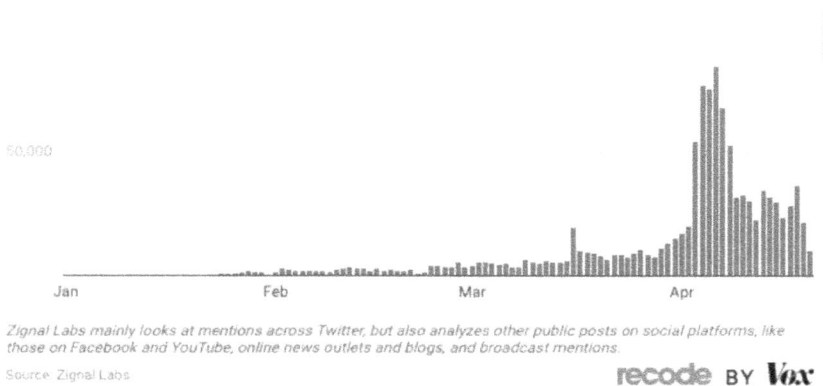

Social media mentions of coronavirus alongside 5G took off this spring

50,000

Jan   Feb   Mar   Apr

Zignal Labs mainly looks at mentions across Twitter, but also analyzes other public posts on social platforms, like those on Facebook and YouTube, online news outlets and blogs, and broadcast mentions.

Source: Zignal Labs   recode BY Vox

FIGURE 2: *This graph shows the explosion in online mentions of 5G in relation to COVID-19 in 2020 (**Heilweil, 2020**)*

As Heilweil (2020) reported, these theories have circulated due to several anti-5G Facebook communities, like "Lawful Stop5G Rebellion No Violence", with 35,000 members. Furthermore, this theory spread like wildfire when celebrities like Wiz Khalifa, Woody Harrelson, and Keri Hilton have posted about it. While this conspiracy seems outlandish, it has damaging consequences as it sows mistrust in public health experts. Moreover, it makes the pandemic look like a technological hoax. When this theory circulated at its peak in April 2020, it led to cell towers being burnt down in Britain (Satariano & Alba, 2020).

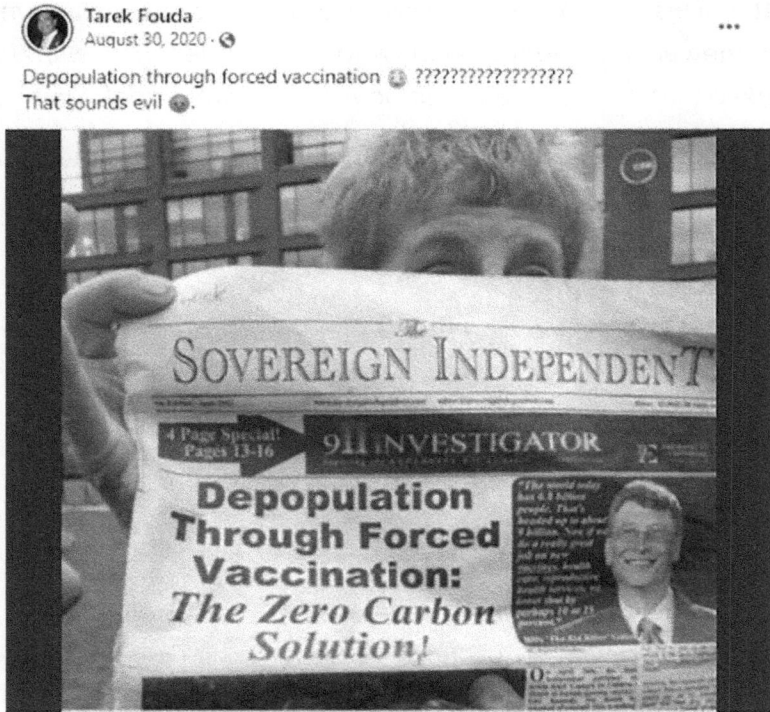

Tarek Fouda
August 30, 2020 · ⊙

Depopulation through forced vaccination 🤨 ???????????????????
That sounds evil 😠.

FIGURE 3: *This image shows a 2011 article from a local newspaper circulated through social media and the internet as a means to illustrate the theory that the pandemic was planned. However, this theory was debunked (AAP FactCheck, 2021)*

Another popular theory that has populated the internet is that vaccines are a solution to reducing overpopulation. For instance, Figure 3 shows an image from an Irish newspaper that takes Bill Gates out of context when he said, *"new vaccines, health care, and reproductive services may reduce population growth"*. This was taken from a TED Talk on reducing global emissions, citing the common trend that as health services and vaccination rates increase, population growth decreases. This was due to the idea that parents would not need large families as they would be confident that their children would survive to adulthood (*AAP FactCheck, 2021*). Taking this quote out of context allowed for it to be misconstrued and twisted, where it is implied that vaccinations will be used to kill people directly.

While these theories can seem outlandish to some, they illustrate the lack of public health education in parts of the world. The spread of these damaging conspiracies is not based on malicious intent—but a strong fear of the unknown and mistrust of higher authorities. In response, many organizations are pushing for stricter measures to regulate social media and stop the spread of these theories in their tracks. This brings up an important question—Where do we draw the line between spreading misinformation and free speech? Taking away the stage upon which these conspiracies circulate, whether it be Twitter, Instagram, Facebook, is only a temporary solution to a very real problem. A lack of public health literacy and education and a general mistrust in government and authority create these attitudes. Rather than pausing and looking further into a sensationalized theory spread through an unreliable source, several individuals believe in these theories as it confirms their current attitudes of mistrust in governments and health authorities. Many organizations like the World Health Organization are attacking this problem by trying to increase public health education through online initiatives like Mythbusters where they break down popular COVID-19 myths. However, it can easily fall onto deaf ears as individuals who simply have mistrust in public health authorities will simply ignore these initiatives. It may also be beneficial for senior health officials to directly engage with large anti-vaccine communities online (for example live interviews or AMAs) to address certain myths and issues. While this is easier said than done, it can present new perspectives and break down the echo chamber where anti-vaccine sentiment festers continuously.

Conspiracy Theories connected to Religious Beliefs

Vaccines are the Antichrist

Many conspiracy theories have been created as a result of strong religious beliefs. As Dwoskin (*2021*) reported, the coronavirus vaccine was considered by some to be "the biblical End Time". Furthermore, false theories regarding vaccines populate niche parts of social media—such as the idea that they contain fetal tissue and are associated with the devil. On Tiktok, Christians pretended to be forced to take the vaccine, to later smear blood on themselves and pretend to die (*Dwoskin, 2021*). Some Christian influencers and ministries have also joined the cause, spreading misinformation that the vaccines contained ingredients that are "the mark of the beast", a biblical reference to when the Antichrist asked Christians to put a mark on their bodies. These theories contribute to the high vaccine hesitancy rates among certain religious demographics.

Americans' intentions to get a COVID-19 vaccine

% U.S. adults

	Will definitely/probably get a vaccine for COVID-19, or have already gotten at least one dose (NET)	Received at least one vaccine dose	Definitely/Probably will get a vaccine	Definitely/Probably will NOT get a vaccine for COVID-19	No answer
Protestant	62	19	44	36	1
White evangelical	54	17	37	45	1
White, not evangelical	72	25	48	27	1
Black Protestant	64	17	47	33	2
Catholic	77	23	54	22	1
White	78	27	51	21	1
Hispanic	77	15	61	22	2
Unaffiliated	71	16	55	28	1
Atheist	90	20	70	10	<1
Agnostic	80	17	62	20	<1
Nothing in particular	64	14	49	36	1

Source: Survey conducted Feb. 16-21, 2021.
"Growing Share of Americans Say They Plan To Get a COVID-19 Vaccine – or Already Have"

PEW RESEARCH CENTER

FIGURE 4: *In a Pew research study analyzing 10,121 US adults, White Evangelicals along with Black Protestants have the highest rates of refusing the vaccine (**Funk & Tyson, 2021**).*

45% of White evangelicals along with 33% of Black protestants said they definitely/probably were not going to take the vaccine—this is some of the highest anti-vaccine sentiments recorded among any demographic. Anti-science and conspiracy theories have historically affected certain religious demographics. According to Fea, a historian with expertise in evangelism, "it goes back to the Scopes trial" where the theory of evolution was debated by evangelicals. Additionally, there is also distrust in vaccine science as there is a strong "belief that God will protect them" (*Shimran, 2021*).

African Americans are also particularly vulnerable to vaccine hesitancy due to their mistrust having historical roots of mistreatment and abuse (*Williams, 2021*). The Henrietta Lacks case is an example of a black women's cancer tumor sampled without her consent. Next, the Tuskegee research experiment in the 1930s saw health officials ignoring syphilis in black men as a way to observe the disease (*Williams, 2021*). Furthermore, some research is even suggesting that this discrepancy in health treatment is even present today. One study that analyzed 67,487 patients found that opioids were less likely to be prescribed to Blacks and that this disparity was especially present for conditions with fewer objective findings like migraines (*Tamayo-Sarver et al., 2003*). While more studies on discrimination in the health setting need to be performed to form a concrete conclusion, it is clear that there are strong historic roots of mistreatment—which could be present today as well. This has resulted in some mistrust in health professionals. In fact, one peer-reviewed study analyzed 527 African Americans and 382 white respondents, to find that 45.5% of African Americans *"believed their physicians exposed them to unnecessary risks"* compared to 34.8% of white respondents (*Corbie-Smith, 2002*). These are staggering statistics that suggest that there is mistrust in public health authorities, to varying extents.

This may contribute to the high vaccine hesitancy and the incli-nation to believe in conspiracy theories (ex: vaccines contain "the mark of the beast") that are not backed by evidence. There is a strong propensity to also spread these theories that validate their fears and mistrust. Additionally, they can connect with other like-minded individuals who have similar anti-vaccine attitudes. This fear of public health authorities and government has historic roots that need to be addressed to strengthen vaccination efforts.

Vaccines contain gelatin/pork products

In another case, another common theory regarding COVID-19 vaccines is that they contain gelatin or products related to pork. This makes the vaccines non-kosher for Jews and also haram or forbidden for Muslims as well. A survey was conducted in partnership with the World Health Organization (WHO) and the Ministry of Health in Indonesia, the country with the high-est number of Muslims. It found that 27% of respondents were hesitant to take the vaccine (*Al Jazeera, 2021a*). While vaccines for other diseases have used gelatin in the past, this theory was debunked, as all COVID-19 vaccines are completely pork/gelatin-free (*Hope, 2021*). This problem is not unique only to Indonesia but to all countries with sizable Muslim populations like the U.K where Imams (Muslim leaders) and influencers have united to quell vaccine fears (*Al Jezeera, 2021b*). Various task forces have been formed globally to address this issue of misinformation—like the Canadian Muslim COVID-19 Task Force made of health experts and religious leaders (Rodriguez, 2021). In another case, 70 Jewish doctors signed an open letter to publicly address common vaccine myths (*Rashty, 2020*). Orga-nizations and initiatives like these are powerful in disarming anti-vaccine sentiment as individuals already within religious communities are better equipped to properly addressing concerns of people with vaccine concerns.

Closing Discussion and Solutions

A common theme persists in all of these conspiracy theories. The prevalence of these theories is rooted in a mistrust in public health authorities and government. Furthermore, there could also be a lack of knowledge or a strong fear of the unknown like new technology. All of these factors can lead individuals to believe in conspiracy theories that simply affirm their fears and mistrust.

These theories can most likely never be eliminated. There will likely always be individuals that will believe in baseless theories. A more realistic focus can be placed on trying to stop the rapid spread of these attitudes. A global education effort is underway to stop misinformation in the age of the internet. Essential skills like assessing trustworthy sources, evaluating evidence, and rejecting misinformation are all essential skills that can not only stop the spread of COVID-19 vaccine conspiracies but conspiracy theories of all sorts. These skills will not only build a more analytical population but one that scrutinizes all information presented to them. All agents, including public health authorities and governments, will have to meet high standards to meet the scrutiny of an educated population. Deeper roots of mistrust in specific demographics like members of certain religions require a greater strategic effort to help solve these issues. Influential organizations within these demographics can help build trust. Having productive conversations where these fears and concerns can directly be addressed will be especially useful in breaking down persistent echo chambers and strengthening vaccination campaigns.

All in all, solutions like taking away social media platforms where these theories exist are simply a band-aid as they stop the spread of the conspiracy temporarily. Attacking the root issues of fear and mistrust will be a much more permanent solution.

Conclusion

Ivy Truong

THE COVID-19 PANDEMIC has taken a toll on every aspect of the globe, leaving no nation untouched. With up to 700,000 new cases daily (*World Health Organization, 2020*), the transmission of coronavirus does not seem to be slowing down. It is crucial that a vaccine is developed and distributed globally to ensure that the spread of the virus is quieted to a controllable state. A major problem with this is that conventional vaccine development platforms cannot provide the rapid development that is required in the current situation. This is more common than expected, many infectious pathogens that have resulted in pandemics for which no effective vaccines have been developed, such as tuberculosis, and the Human Immunodeficiency Virus (HIV) (*Gebre et al., 2021*). This reflects the historical commonality that generally, pandemics were not halted by the introduction of vaccines. Instead, other ways to combat past pandemics were implemented, such as simple public health measures (as in the case with SARS-CoV1) or antiretroviral therapy (as with HIV). Each pandemic was halted by using the disease's characteristics, such as with SARS-CoV1 where the pathogen was most transmissible when the patients were sick, thus isolation in the appearance of those symptoms effectively reduced the further infection to a great extent. With regards to COVID-19, the proportion of asymptomatic (here it is defined as "a laboratory-confirmed infected person without overt symptoms" (*WHO, 2020*) infection ranges from 18% to 81% (*Nikolai, et al., 2020*), signifying that isolation of symptoms is much more difficult in this case. The COVID-19 pandemic is driven by asymptomatic infections, demonstratively, 41% of the population in Vo, the first Italian city with a confirmed death, were asymptomatic before the lockdown (*Nikolai, et al., 2020*). This explains the difficulty in controlling the infectious rate despite its lack of overt and deadly symptoms. The range of symptoms that the disease covers provides an answer as to why lessons from previous pandemics cannot be fully implemented here, pointing to the greater emphasis on vaccines as the means of stopping the pandemic.

The solution to confronting the highly infectious SARS-CoV2 is the development of mRNA vaccines, a new vaccine platform that drastically shortens the 10-15 year time span normally required for vaccine development. The goal of implementing a vaccine programme in a pandemic is to confer herd immunity, whereby a large portion of the population becomes immune to the disease to reduce the transmission of the virus. By utilizing the body's protein synthesis mechanisms, there is no need for pathogen growth, harvest, and testing, instead, the body synthesizes the very antigen that induces the body's immune response. mRNA vaccine design has been in progress, with many breakthroughs for the last decade, but the coronavirus provided momentum for the synthesis of the mRNA vaccines and most importantly, became the disease target that allowed for comparison between the different mRNA vaccine candidates (*Verbecke et al., 2020*). Approval of the revolutionary mRNA vaccines Moderna and Pfizer-BioNtech alongside the traditional vaccines Sputnik and AstraZeneca gives rise to a tremendously informative case study on the various vaccine development strategies and allows for further optimization of future vaccine development.

The revolutionary development of mRNA vaccines provides a ray of hope for a near end of the pandemic, however, it is important to also shift our attention on the importance of vaccine distribution, which is impeded by many factors. A component seen in previous pandemics is the shortage of vaccines in countries with developing health care systems, usually caused by production monopoly, complex distribution processes, and reduced producers (*Jacobsen et al., 2007*). Another large component that has grown to a substantial amount is vaccine hesitancy, which increased drastically to a worrying extent during the COVID-19 pandemic. Vaccine hesitancy ranging from misinformation or a lack of information on the new vaccine developments to outlandish beliefs concerning vaccines and the disease as a whole greatly impedes the mass immunization required for acquiring herd immunity. The reasons for vaccine hesitancy are complex and contextual, requiring personalized means of addressing them for different demographics. The overall goal, however, is to change the perceptions of vaccines and the coronavirus through vaccine programmes. With the increasing spread of misinformation, the platforms used for the communication of the misinformation must be seized and utilized in a manner that promotes accurate information systems about immunizations. For the pandemic to truly end, we must not rely on vaccine research alone, rather, focusing on social factors and information programmes aids in slowing down the infection and preventing new variants from emerging.

With the approval for distribution of various COVID-19 vaccines increasing, the long-awaited end of the pandemic looms near. While we patiently wait for the population to become immunized, we should not forget to continue implementing the public safety measures such as physically distancing and wearing a mask to prevent spreading the virus as best we can, and playing a supporting role for the vaccines to accomplish the goal for herd immunity, effectively ending the pandemic and stopping the transmission of the coronavirus. With the groundbreaking development of mRNA vaccines and vaccine hesitancy now serving as a threat against mass immunizations, the importance of vaccines is emphasized in the COVID-19 pandemic more than it has ever before.

Bibliography

Introduction

CDC. (2020, April 2). *COVID-19 and your health.* Centers for Disease Control and Prevention; U.S. Department of Health & Human Services. https://www.cdc.gov/coronavirus/2019-ncov/transmission/variant.html

Corbett, K. S., Edwards, D. K., Leist, S. R., Abiona, O. M., Boyoglu-Barnum, S., Gillespie, R. A., Himansu, S., Schäfer, A., Ziwawo, C. T., DiPiazza, A. T., Dinnon, K. H., Elbashir, S. M., Shaw, C. A., Woods, A., Fritch, E. J., Martinez, D. R., Bock, K. W., Minai, M., Nagata, B. M., & Hutchinson, G. B. (2020). SARS-CoV-2 mRNA vaccine design enabled by prototype pathogen preparedness. *Nature*, 586(7830), 567–571. https://doi.org/10.1038/s41586-020-2622-0

Douglas, K. M., Sutton, R. M., & Cichocka, A. (2017). The psychology of conspiracy theories. *Current Directions in Psychological Science*, 26(6), 538–542. https://doi.org/10.1177/0963721417718261

How Vaccines Are Made | History of Vaccines. (2000). The History of Vaccines; The College of Physicians of Philadelphia. https://www.historyofvaccines.org/content/how-vaccines-are-made

Mills, M., Rahal, C., Brazel, D., Yan, J., & Gieysztor, S. (2020). *COVID-19 vaccine deployment: Behaviour, ethics, misinformation and policy strategies.* Social Science in Humanitarian Action Platform; IDS, UNICEF, Wellcome Trust & FCDO. https://www.socialscienceinaction.org/resources/covid-19-vaccine-deployment-behaviour-ethics-misinformation-and-policy-strategies/

Ramirez, V. B., & Biggers, A. (2020, April 20). *What is R0? Gauging contagious infections.* Healthline. https://www.healthline.com/health/r-nought-reproduction-number#covid-19-r-0

Randolph, H. E., & Barreiro, L. B. (2020). Herd immunity: Understanding COVID-19. *Immunity*, 52(5), 737–741. https://doi.org/10.1016/j.immuni.2020.04.012

Ullah, I., Khan, K. S., Tahir, M. J., Ahmed, A., & Harapan, H. (2021). Myths and conspiracy theories on vaccines and COVID-19: Potential effect on global vaccine refusals. *Vacunas*. https://doi.org/10.1016/j.vacun.2021.01.001

Verbeke, R., Lentacker, I., & Smedt, S. C. D. (2021). The dawn of mRNA vaccines: The COVID-19 case. *Journal of Controlled Release*, 333, 511–520. https://doi.org/10.1016/j.jconrel.2021.03.043

Zhang, L., Jackson, C. B., Mou, H., Ojha, A., Rangarajan, E. S., Izard, T., Farzan, M., & Choe, H. (2020). The D614G mutation in the SARS-CoV-2 spike protein reduces S1 shedding and increases infectivity. *BioRxiv*. https://doi.org/10.1101/2020.06.12.148726

Chapter 1

Boylston, A. (2012). *The origins of inoculation. Journal of the Royal Society of Medicine*, 105(7), 309-313. https://doi.org/10.1258/jrsm.2012.12k044

Britannica. (n.d.). *History of medicine*. Encyclopedia Britannica. Retrieved May 3, 2021, from https://www.britannica.com/science/history-of-medicine/

Canadian Public Health Association. (n.d.). *The story of polio*. https://www.cpha.ca/story-polio#:-:text=An%20estimated%2011%2C000%20people%20in,with%20nearly%202%2C000%20paralytic%20cases.

Centers for Disease Control and Prevention. (2021, March 4). *Understanding mRNA COVID-19 vaccines*. https://www.cdc.gov/coronavirus/2019-ncov/vaccines/different-vaccines/mrna.html

The College of Physicians of Philadelphia. (n.d.). *Timeline*. The history of vaccines. Retrieved May 3, 2021, from https://www.historyofvaccines.org/timeline#EVT_100514

Fitzpatrick, M. (2006). The Cutter incident: How America's first Polio vaccine led to a growing vaccine crisis. *Journal of the Royal Society of Medicine*, 99(3), 156.

Hoyt, K. (2006). Vaccine innovation: Lessons from World War II. *Journal of Public Health Policy*, 27, 38-57. https://doi.org/10.1057/palgrave.jphp.3200064

Jiang, S., He, Y., & Liu, S. (2005). SARS vaccine development. *Emerging Infectious Diseases, 11*(7), 1016-1020. https://doi.org/10.3201/eid1107.05021

Kurlander, C., & Juhl, R. P. (2020, September 26). *Lessons from how the polio vaccine went from the lab to the public that Americans can learn from today.* ASBMB Today. https://www.asbmb.org/asbmb-today/science/092620/lessons-from-how-the-polio-vaccine-went-from-the-l

Li, Y.D., Chi, W.Y., Su, J.H., Ferrall, L., & Hung, C.F. (2020). Coronavirus vaccine development: from SARS and MERS to COVID-19. *Journal of Biomedical Science*, 27, 104. https://doi.org/10.1186/s12929-020-00695-2

Padron-Regalado, E. (2020). Vaccines for SARS-CoV-2: Lessons from other coronavirus strains. *Infectious Diseases and Therapy*, 9(2), 255-274. https://doi.org/10.1007/s40121-020-00300-x

Pardi, N., Hogan, M. J., Porter, F. W., & Weissman, D. (2018). mNRA vaccines – A new era in vaccinology. *Nature Reviews Drug Discovery*, 17, 261-279. https://doi.org/10.1038/nrd.2017.243

Riedel, S. (2005). Edward Jenner and the history of smallpox and vaccination. *Baylor University Medical Center Proceedings*, 18(1), 21-25. https://doi.org/10.1080/08998280.2005.11928028

Roossinck, M. J. (2020, May 5). *The mysterious disappearance of the first SARS virus, and why we need a vaccine for the current one but didn't for the other.* The Conversation. https://theconversation.com/the-mysterious-disappearance-of-the-first-sars-virus-and-why-we-need-a-vaccine-for-the-current-one-but-didnt-for-the-other-137583

Sanders, B., Koldijk, M., & Schuitemaker, H. (2014). Inactivated viral vaccines. *Vaccine Analysis: Strategies, Principles, and Control*, 45–80. https://doi.org/10.1007/978-3-662-45024-6_2

Schlake, T., Thess, A., Fotin-Mleczek, M., & Kallen, K. J. (2012). Developing mRNA-vaccine technologies. *RNA Biology*, 9(11), 1319–1330. https://doi.org/10.4161/rna.22269

Watts, E. (2020, April 28). *What Rome learned from the deadly Antonine Plague of 165 A.D.* Smithsonian Magazine. https://www.smithsonianmag.com/history/what-rome-learned-deadly-antonine-plague-165-d-180974758/

Wever, P. C., & van Bergen, L. (2012). Prevention of tetanus during the First World War. *Medical Humanities*, 38(2), 78-82. doi: 10.1136/medhum-2011-010157

World Health Organisation (n.d.). *Smallpox*. Retrieved May 4, 2021, from https://www.who.int/health-topics/smallpox#tab=tab_1

Zhang, C., Maruggi, G., Shan, H., & Li, J. (2019). Advances in mRNA vaccines for infectious diseases. *Frontiers in Immunology*, 10(594). doi: 10.3389/fimmu.2019.00594

Chapter 2

ALIMOHAMADI, Y., SEPANDI, M., TAGHDIR, M., & HOSAMIRUD-SARI, H. (2020). Determine the most common clinical symptoms in COVID-19 patients: A systematic review and meta-analysis. *Journal of Preventive Medicine and Hygiene*, 61(3), E304–E312. https://doi.org/10.15167/2421-4248/jpmh2020.61.3.1530

Arslan, M., Xu, B., & Gamal El-Din, M. (2020). Transmission of SARS-CoV-2 via fecal-oral and aerosols–borne routes: Environmental dynamics and implications for wastewater management in underprivileged societies. *The Science of the Total Environment*, 743, 140709. https://doi.org/10.1016/j.scitotenv.2020.140709

Canada, H. (2021, February 26). AstraZeneca / COVISHIELD COVID-19 vaccine: What you should know [Education and awareness]. *Aem.*

https://www.canada.ca/en/health-canada/services/drugs-health-products/covid19-industry/drugs-vaccines-treatments/vaccines/astrazeneca.html

Canada, P. H. A. of. (2020, November 3). The facts about COVID-19 vaccines [Education and awareness]. *Aem*. https://www.canada.ca/en/public-health/services/diseases/2019-novel-coronavirus-infection/awareness-resources/know-vaccine.html

CDC. (2020a, February 11). Coronavirus Disease 2019 (COVID-19). *Centers for Disease Control and Prevention*. https://www.cdc.gov/coronavirus/2019-ncov/cdcresponse/about-COVID-19.html

CDC. (2020b, February 11). Coronavirus Disease 2019 (COVID-19). *Centers for Disease Control and Prevention*. https://www.cdc.gov/coronavirus/2019-ncov/more/science-and-research/surface-transmission.html

Ciotti, M., Angeletti, S., Minieri, M., Giovannetti, M., Benvenuto, D., Pascarella, S., Sagnelli, C., Bianchi, M., Bernardini, S., & Ciccozzi, M. (2019). COVID-19 Outbreak: An Overview. *Chemotherapy*, 64(5–6), 215–223. https://doi.org/10.1159/000507423

Coronavirus disease (COVID-19). (n.d.-a). Retrieved May 5, 2021, from https://www.who.int/news-room/q-a-detail/coronavirus-disease-covid-19

Coronavirus disease (COVID-19): How is it transmitted? (n.d.-b). Retrieved May 4, 2021, from https://www.who.int/news-room/q-a-detail/coronavirus-disease-covid-19-how-is-it-transmitted

Coronavirus: What is it and how can I protect myself? *Mayo Clinic*. (n.d.). Retrieved May 4, 2021, from https://www.mayoclinic.org/diseases-conditions/coronavirus/expert-answers/novel-coronavirus/faq-20478727

COVID-19: Here are the questions about the virus we still can't answer. (2020, May 19). *Coronavirus*. https://www.ctvnews.ca/health/coronavirus/covid-19-here-are-the-questions-about-the-virus-we-still-can-t-answer-1.4944990

COVID-19 Routes of Transmission – What We Know So Far. (n.d.). 44.

COVID-19 Variants of Concern (VOCs). (n.d.). Public Health Ontario. Retrieved May 3, 2021, from https://www.publichealthontario.ca/ Diseases and Conditions/Infectious Diseases/Respiratory Diseases/Novel Coronavirus/Variants

Get the facts about COVID-19 vaccines. (n.d.). *Mayo Clinic.* Retrieved May 6, 2021, from https://www.mayoclinic.org/diseases-conditions/coronavirus/ in-depth/coronavirus-vaccine/art-20484859

Hu, B., Guo, H., Zhou, P., & Shi, Z.-L. (2021). Characteristics of SARS-CoV-2 and COVID-19. *Nature Reviews Microbiology*, 19(3), 141–154. https:// doi.org/10.1038/s41579-020-00459-7

Hu, J., & Wang, Y. (2021). The Clinical Characteristics and Risk Factors of Severe COVID-19. *Gerontology*, 1–12. https://doi.org/10.1159/000513400

Khanna, R. C., Cicinelli, M. V., Gilbert, S. S., Honavar, S. G., & Murthy, G. V. S. (2020). COVID-19 pandemic: Lessons learned and future directions. *Indian Journal of Ophthalmology*, 68(5), 703–710. https://doi.org/10.4103/ijo. IJO_843_20

Li, H., Liu, S.-M., Yu, X.-H., Tang, S.-L., & Tang, C.-K. (2020). Coronavirus disease 2019 (COVID-19): Current status and future perspectives. *International Journal of Antimicrobial Agents*, 55(5), 105951. https://doi.org/10.1016/j. ijantimicag.2020.105951

Mallapaty, S. (2021). Where did COVID come from? Five mysteries that remain. *Nature,* 591(7849), 188–189. https://doi.org/10.1038/ d41586-021-00502-4

Maragakis, L. L. (2020). Eye Protection and the Risk of Coronavirus Disease 2019: Does Wearing Eye Protection Mitigate Risk in Public, Non–Health Care Settings? *JAMA Ophthalmology*, 138(11), 1199. https://doi. org/10.1001/jamaophthalmol.2020.3909

Mayo Clinic Staff. (n.d.). COVID-19: Who's at higher risk of serious symptoms? *Mayo Clinic*. Retrieved May 5, 2021, from https://www.mayoclinic.org/diseases-conditions/coronavirus/in-depth/coronavirus-who-is-at-risk/art-20483301

Moore, J. P., & Offit, P. A. (2021). SARS-CoV-2 Vaccines and the Growing Threat of Viral Variants. *JAMA*, 325(9), 821. https://doi.org/10.1001/jama.2021.1114

New Variants of Coronavirus: What You Should Know. (n.d.). Retrieved May 3, 2021, from https://www.hopkinsmedicine.org/health/conditions-and-diseases/coronavirus/a-new-strain-of-coronavirus-what-you-should-know

Roberts, J. D., Dickinson, K. L., Koebele, E., Neuberger, L., Banacos, N., Blanch-Hartigan, D., Welton-Mitchell, C., & Birkland, T. A. (2020). Clinicians, cooks, and cashiers: Examining health equity and the COVID-19 risks to essential workers. *Toxicology and Industrial Health*, 36(9), 689–702. https://doi.org/10.1177/0748233720970439

Scudellari, M. (2020). How the pandemic might play out in 2021 and beyond. *Nature*, 584(7819), 22–25. https://doi.org/10.1038/d41586-020-02278-5

Tosh, P. K. (n.d.). COVID-19: How can I protect myself? *Mayo Clinic*. Retrieved May 2, 2021, from https://www.mayoclinic.org/diseases-conditions/coronavirus/expert-answers/novel-coronavirus/faq-20478727

Chapter 3

Arif, T. B. (2021). The 501.V2 and B.1.1.7 variants of coronavirus disease 2019 (COVID-19): A new time-bomb in the making? *Infection Control & Hospital Epidemiology*, 1–2. https://doi.org/10.1017/ice.2020.1434

Barr, J. N., & Fearns, R. (2016). Genetic Instability of RNA Viruses. *Genome Stability*, 21–35. https://doi.org/10.1016B978-0-12-803309-8.00002-1

Caspermeyer, J. (2016). When Silent Mutations Provide Evolutionary Advantages. *Molecular Biology and Evolution*, 33(6), 1639.2-1639. https://doi.org/10.1093/molbev/msw078

Duffy, S. (2018). Why are RNA virus mutation rates so damn high? *PLOS Biology*, 16(8), e3000003. https://doi.org/10.1371/journal.pbio.3000003

Galloway, S. E. (2021). Emergence of SARS-CoV-2 B.1.1.7 Lineage — United States, December 29, 2020–January 12, 2021. MMWR. *Morbidity and Mortality Weekly Report*, 70(3). https://doi.org/10.15585/mmwr.mm7003e2

Madzokere, E., & Herrero, L. (2021). *What's the difference between mutations, variants and strains? A guide to COVID terminology.* The Conversation. Retrieved May 7, 2021, from https://theconversation.com/whats-the-difference-between-mutations-variants-and-strains-a-guide-to-covid-terminology-154825#:~:text=A%20variant%20is%20referred%20to%20as%20a%20strain

Mutations are random. (2021). Berkeley.edu. https://evolution.berkeley.edu/evolibrary/article/mutations_07#:~:text=The%20Lederberg%20experiment%20In%201952%2C%20Esther%20and%20Joshua

Quack, N. (2021, January 4). *Science Blog: S-Gene Target Failure is Proxy for VOC 202012/01 COVID-19 strain.* Science Blog. https://sciencereject.blogspot.com/2021/01/s-gene-target-failure-is-proxy-for-voc.html#:~:text=This%20is%20called%20S-Gene%20Target%20Failure%2C%20or%20simply

Rabaan, A., Al-Ahmed, S., Haque, S., Sah, R., Tiwari, R., Singh Malik, Y., Dhama, K., Yatoo, M., Katterine Bonilla-Aldana, D., Rodriguez-Morales, A., & And Kashmir, J. (n.d.). *SARS-CoV-2, SARS-CoV, and MERS-CoV: a comparative overview.*

Standl, F., Jöckel, K.-H., Brune, B., Schmidt, B., & Stang, A. (2020). Comparing SARS-CoV-2 with SARS-CoV and influenza pandemics. *The Lancet Infectious Diseases.* https://doi.org/10.1016/s1473-3099(20)30648-4

Steinhauer, D. A., Domingo, E., & Holland, J. J. (1992). Lack of evidence for proofreading mechanisms associated with an RNA virus polymerase. Gene, 122(2), 281–288. https://doi.org/10.1016/0378-1119(92)90216-c

The Origins of SARS-CoV-2 | Science-Based Medicine. (2021, March 31). Sciencebasedmedicine.org. https://sciencebasedmedicine.org/

the-origins-of-sars-cov-2/

Visser, J. A. G. M., Hermisson, J., Wagner, G. P., Meyers, L. A., Bagheri Chaichian, H., Blanchard, J. L., Chao, L., Cheverud, J. M., Elena, S. F., Fontana, W., Gibson, G., Hansen, T. F., Krakauer, D., Lewontin, R. C., Ofria, C., Rice, S. H., Dassow, G. von, Wagner, A., & Whitlock, M. C. (2003). PERSPECTIVE: EVOLUTION AND DETECTION OF GENETIC ROBUSTNESS. *Evolution*, 57(9), 1959–1972. https://doi.org/10.1111/j.0014-3820.2003.tb00377.x

How Many Strains of the Coronavirus Are There? About New Variants. (2021, March 12). Healthline. https://www.healthline.com/health/how-many-strains-of-covid-are-there#uk-variant

CDC. (2020, February 11). *Cases, Data, and Surveillance.* Centers for Disease Control and Prevention. https://www.cdc.gov/coronavirus/2019-ncov/cases-updates/variant-surveillance/variant-info.html#Interest

SARS-CoV-2 variants of concern as of 6 May 2021. (n.d.). European Centre for Disease Prevention and Control. Retrieved May 7, 2021, from https://www.ecdc.europa.eu/en/covid-19/variants-concern

An EUA for Bamlanivimab—A Monoclonal Antibody for COVID-19. (2020). JAMA. https://doi.org/10.1001/jama.2020.24415

Commissioner, O. of the. (2021, February 9). Coronavirus (COVID-19) Update: FDA Authorizes Monoclonal Antibodies for Treatment of COVID-19. FDA. https://www.fda.gov/news-events/press-announcements/coronavirus-covid-19-update-fda-authorizes-monoclonal-antibodies-treatment-covid-19-0

Davies, N. G., Abbott, S., Barnard, R. C., Jarvis, C. I., Kucharski, A. J., Munday, J. D., Pearson, C. A. B., Russell, T. W., Tully, D. C., Washburne, A. D., Wenseleers, T., Gimma, A., Waites, W., Wong, K. L. M., van Zandvoort, K., Silverman, J. D., Diaz-Ordaz, K., Keogh, R., Eggo, R. M., & Funk, S. (2021). Estimated transmissibility and impact of SARS-CoV-2 lineage B.1.1.7 in England. Science, eabg3055. https://doi.org/10.1126/science.abg3055

FACT SHEET FOR HEALTH CARE PROVIDERS EMERGENCY
USE AUTHORIZATION (EUA) OF BAMLANIVIMAB AND ETESE-
VIMAB AUTHORIZED USE. (n.d.). https://www.fda.gov/media/145802/
download

FACT SHEET FOR HEALTH CARE PROVIDERS EMERGENCY
USE AUTHORIZATION (EUA) OF REGEN-COV TM (casirivimab
with imdevimab). (n.d.). Retrieved May 8, 2021, from https://www.fda.gov/
media/145611/download

Graham, M. S., Sudre, C. H., May, A., Antonelli, M., Murray, B., Varsavsky,
T., Kläser, K., Canas, L. S., Molteni, E., Modat, M., Drew, D. A., Nguyen,
L. H., Polidori, L., Selvachandran, S., Hu, C., Capdevila, J., Hammers, A.,
Chan, A. T., Wolf, J., & Spector, T. D. (2021). Changes in symptomatology, reinfection, and transmissibility associated with the SARS-CoV-2
variant B.1.1.7: an ecological study. The Lancet Public Health. https://doi.
org/10.1016/s2468-2667(21)00055-4

Jangra, S., Ye, C., Rathnasinghe, R., Stadlbauer, D., Krammer, F., Simon,
V., Martinez-Sobrido, L., García-Sastre, A., Schotsaert, M., Alshammary,
H., Amoako, A. A., Awawda, M. H., Beach, K. F., Bermúdez-González,
M. C., Chernet, R. L., Eaker, L. Q., Ferreri, E. D., Floda, D. L., Gleason,
C. R., & Kleiner, G. (2021). SARS-CoV-2 spike E484K mutation reduces
antibody neutralisation. The Lancet Microbe. https://doi.org/10.1016/
s2666-5247(21)00068-9

Planas, D., Bruel, T., Grzelak, L., Guivel-Benhassine, F., Staropoli, I.,
Porrot, F., Planchais, C., Buchrieser, J., Rajah, M. M., Bishop, E., Albert,
M., Donati, F., Prot, M., Behillil, S., Enouf, V., Maquart, M., Smati-Lafarge,
M., Varon, E., Schortgen, F., & Yahyaoui, L. (2021). Sensitivity of infectious
SARS-CoV-2 B.1.1.7 and B.1.351 variants to neutralizing antibodies. Nature
Medicine. https://doi.org/10.1038/s41591-021-01318-5

Wang, P., Liu, L., Iketani, S., Luo, Y., Guo, Y., Wang, M., Yu, J., Zhang,
B., Kwong, P. D., Graham, B. S., Mascola, J. R., Chang, J. Y., Yin, M.
T., Sobieszczyk, M., Kyratsous, C. A., Shapiro, L., Sheng, Z., Nair, M.
S., Huang, Y., & Ho, D. D. (2021). Increased Resistance of SARS-CoV-2

Variants B.1.351 and B.1.1.7 to Antibody Neutralization. https://doi. org/10.1101/2021.01.25.428137

Wang, P., Wang, M., Yu, J., Cerutti, G., Nair, M. S., Huang, Y., Kwong, P. D., Shapiro, L., & Ho, D. D. (2021). Increased Resistance of SARS-CoV-2 Variant P.1 to Antibody Neutralization. https://doi. org/10.1101/2021.03.01.433466

Yadav, P. D., Sapkal, G. N., Abraham, P., Ella, R., Deshpande, G., Patil, D. Y., Nyayanit, D. A., Gupta, N., Sahay, R. R., Shete, A. M., Panda, S., Bhargava, B., & Mohan, V. K. (2021). Neutralization of variant under investigation B.1.617 with sera of BBV152 vaccinees. https://doi. org/10.1101/2021.04.23.441101

Garcia-Beltran, W. F., Lam, E. C., Denis, K. S., Nitido, A. D., Garcia, Z. H., Hauser, B. M., Feldman, J., Pavlovic, M. N., Gregory, D. J., Poznansky, M. C., Sigal, A., Schmidt, A. G., Iafrate, A. J., Naranbhai, V., & Balazs, A. B. (2021). Multiple SARS-CoV-2 variants escape neutralization by vaccine-induced humoral immunity. *Cell*, 184(9), 2372-2383.e9. https://doi. org/10.1016/j.cell.2021.03.013

SARS-CoV-2 *immunity-escape variants*. (n.d.). Retrieved May 8, 2021, from https://assets.publishing.service.gov.uk/government/uploads/system/ uploads/attachment_data/file/954990/s1015-sars-cov-2-immunity-escape-variants.pdf

Chapter 4

Ali, S., Asaria, M., & Stranges, S. (2020). COVID-19 and inequality: are we all in this together? *Canadian Journal of Public Health*, 111(3), 415-416. doi: 10.17269/s41997-020-00351-0

Benefits of getting a COVID-19 vaccine. (2021). Centers for Disease Control and Prevention. Retrieved 5 May 2021, from https://www.cdc.gov/coronavi-rus/2019-ncov/vaccines/vaccine-benefits.html

Boodoosingh, R., Olayemi, L., & Sam, F. (2020). COVID-19 vaccines: Getting Anti-vaxxers involved in the discussion. *World Development*, 136, 105177. doi: 10.1016/j.worlddev.2020.105177

Chen, W. (2020). Promise and challenges in the development of COVID-19 vaccines. *Human Vaccines & Immunotherapeutics*, 16(11), 2604-2608. doi: 10.1080/21645515.2020.1787067

Coronavirus disease (COVID-19): Vaccines. (2021). World Health Organization. Retrieved 5 May 2021, from https://www.who.int/news-room/q-a-detail/coronavirus-disease-(covid-19)-vaccines#:~:text=The%20COVID%2D19%20vaccines,the%20virus%20if%20exposed

Coronavirus: WHO chief criticises 'shocking' global vaccine divide. (2021). BBC News. Retrieved 8 May 2021, from https://www.bbc.com/news/world-56698854#:~:text=%22There%20remains%20a%20shocking%20imbalance,than%20500%2C%22%20he%20said.

Dodd, R., Pickles, K., Nickel, B., Cvejic, E., Ayre, J., & Batcup, C. et al. (2021). Concerns and motivations about COVID-19 vaccination. *The Lancet Infectious Diseases*, 21(2), 161-163. doi: 10.1016/s1473-3099(20)30926-9

Get the facts about COVID-19 vaccines. (2021). Mayo Clinic. Retrieved 5 May 2021, from https://www.mayoclinic.org/diseases-conditions/coronavirus/in-depth/coronavirus-vaccine/art-20484859

Getting the COVID-19 vaccine. (2021). World Health Organisation. Retrieved 5 May 2021, from https://www.who.int/news-room/feature-stories/detail/getting-the-covid-19-vaccine

Global COVID-19 vaccine access: A snapshot of inequality. (2021). KFF. Retrieved 8 May 2021, from https://www.kff.org/policy-watch/global-covid-19-vaccine-access-snapshot-of-inequality/

Gupta, R., & Morain, S. (2020). Ethical allocation of future COVID-19 vaccines. *Journal of Medical Ethics*, 47(3), 137-141. doi: 10.1136/medethics-2020-106850

Herd immunity and COVID-19 (coronavirus): What you need to know. (2021). Mayo Clinic. Retrieved 5 May 2021, from https://www.mayoclinic.org/diseases-conditions/coronavirus/in-depth/herd-immunity-and-coronavirus/art-20486808#:~:text=Herd%20immunity%20also%20can%20

be,causing%20illness%20or%20resulting%20complications

Mishra, S., Stall, N., Ma, H., Odutayo, A., Kwong, J., & Allen, U. et al. (2021). A Vaccination strategy for Ontario COVID-19 hotspots and essential workers. doi: 10.47326/ocsat.2021.02.26.1.0

Nhamo, G., Chikodzi, D., Kunene, H., & Mashula, N. (2020). COVID-19 vaccines and treatments nationalism: Challenges for low-income countries and the attainment of the SDGs. *Global Public Health*, 16(3), 319-339. doi: 10.1080/17441692.2020.1860249

Schwartz, J. (2020). Evaluating and deploying Covid-19 vaccines — The importance of transparency, scientific integrity, and public trust. *New England Journal of Medicine*, 383(18), 1703-1705. doi: 10.1056/nejmp2026393

Webb Hooper, M., Nápoles, A., & Pérez-Stable, E. (2021). No populations left behind: Vaccine hesitancy and equitable diffusion of effective COVID-19 vaccines. *Journal of General Internal Medicine*. doi: 10.1007/s11606-021-06698-5

Chapter 5

Agapov, E. V., Frolov, I., Lindenbach, B. D., Prágai, B. M., Schlesinger, S., & Rice, C. M. (1998). Noncytopathic Sindbis virus RNA vectors for heterologous gene expression. *Proceedings of the National Academy of Sciences of the United States of America*, 95(22), 12989–12994. https://doi.org/10.1073/pnas.95.22.12989

Arteta, M. Y., Kjellman, T., Bartesaghi, S., Wallin, S., Wu, X., Kvist, A. J., Dabkowska, A., Székely, N., Radulescu, A., Bergenholtz, J., & Lindfors, L. (2018). Successful reprogramming of cellular protein production through mRNA delivered by functionalized lipid nanoparticles. *Proceedings of the National Academy of Sciences*, 115(15), E3351–E3360. https://doi.org/10.1073/pnas.1720542115

Bishop, K. J. M., Wilmer, C. E., Soh, S., & Grzybowski, B. A. (2009). *Nanoscale Forces and Their Uses in Self Assembly—Bishop—2009—Small—Wiley Online Library*. https://onlinelibrary.wiley.com/doi/abs/10.1002/smll.200900358

Buschmann, M. D., Carrasco, M. J., Alishetty, S., Paige, M., Alameh, M. G., & Weissman, D. (2021). Nanomaterial Delivery Systems for mRNA Vaccines. Vaccines, 9(1). https://doi.org/10.3390/vaccines9010065

CDC. (2021, March 4). *Understanding mRNA COVID-19 Vaccines*. Centers for Disease Control and Prevention. https://www.cdc.gov/coronavirus/2019-ncov/vaccines/different-vaccines/mrna.html

COVID-19 vaccines for Ontario. (n.d.). COVID-19 (Coronavirus) in Ontario. Retrieved May 8, 2021, from https://covid-19.ontario.ca/covid-19-vaccines-ontario

Crommelin, D. J. A., Anchordoquy, T. J., Volkin, D. B., Jiskoot, W., & Mastrobattista, E. (2021). Addressing the Cold Reality of mRNA Vaccine Stability. *Journal of Pharmaceutical Sciences*, 110(3), 997–1001. https://doi.org/10.1016/j.xphs.2020.12.006

Development and Licensure of Vaccines to Prevent COVID-19; Guidance for Industry. (n.d.). 24.

Dong, Y., Dorkin, J. R., Wang, W., Chang, P. H., Webber, M. J., Tang, B. C., Yang, J., Abutbul-Ionita, I., Danino, D., DeRosa, F., Heartlein, M., Langer, R., & Anderson, D. G. (2016). *Poly(glycoamidoamine) Brushes Formulated Nanomaterials for Systemic siRNA and mRNA Delivery in Vivo | Nano Letters*. https://pubs.acs.org/doi/abs/10.1021/acs.nanolett.5b02428

Fukuhara, H., Ino, Y., & Todo, T. (2016). Oncolytic virus therapy: A new era of cancer treatment at dawn. *Cancer Science*, 107(10), 1373–1379. https://doi.org/10.1111/cas.13027

Hassan, A. O., Kafai, N. M., Dmitriev, I. P., Fox, J. M., Smith, B. K., Harvey, I. B., Chen, R. E., Winkler, E. S., Wessel, A. W., Case, J. B., Kashentseva, E., McCune, B. T., Bailey, A. L., Zhao, H., VanBlargan, L. A., Dai, Y.-N., Ma, M., Adams, L. J., Shrihari, S., … Diamond, M. S. (2020). A Single-Dose Intranasal ChAd Vaccine Protects Upper and Lower Respiratory Tracts against SARS-CoV-2. Cell, 183(1), 169-184.e13. https://doi.org/10.1016/j.cell.2020.08.026

Hoerr, I., Obst, R., Rammensee, H.-G., & Jung, G. (2000). *In vivo application of RNA leads to induction of specific cytotoxic T lymphocytes and antibodies—Hoerr—2000—European Journal of Immunology—Wiley Online Library.* https://onlinelibrary.wiley.com/doi/abs/10.1002/1521-4141(200001)30:1%3C1::AID-IMMU1%3E3.0.CO;2-%23

Jackson, L. A., Anderson, E. J., Rouphael, N. G., & Roberts, P. C. (2020). An mRNA Vaccine against SARS-CoV-2—Preliminary Report | NEJM. *New England Journal of Medicine.* http://www.nejm.org/doi/10.1056/NEJMoa2022483

Jackson, N. A. C., Kester, K. E., Casimiro, D., Gurunathan, S., & DeRosa, F. (2020). The promise of mRNA vaccines: A biotech and industrial perspective. *Npj Vaccines*, 5(1), 1–6. https://doi.org/10.1038/s41541-020-0159-8

Jones, K. L., Drane, D., & Gowans, E. J. (2018). *Long-term storage of DNA-free RNA for use in vaccine studies* | BioTechniques. https://www.future-science.com/doi/full/10.2144/000112593

Kaczmarek, J. C., Patel, A. K., Kauffman, K. J., Fenton, O. S., Webber, M. J., Heartlein, M. W., DeRosa, F., & Anderson, D. G. (2016). Polymer–Lipid Nanoparticles for Systemic Delivery of mRNA to the Lungs. *Angewandte Chemie*, 128(44), 14012–14016. https://doi.org/10.1002/ange.201608450

Kim, J., Eygeris, Y., Gupta, M., & Sahay, G. (2021). Self-assembled mRNA vaccines. *Advanced Drug Delivery Reviews*, 170, 83–112. https://doi.org/10.1016/j.addr.2020.12.014

Krammer, F., Srivastava, K., Alshammary, H., Amoako, A. A., Awawda, M. H., Beach, K. F., Bermúdez-González, M. C., Bielak, D. A., Carreño, J. M., Chernet, R. L., Eaker, L. Q., Ferreri, E. D., Floda, D. L., Gleason, C. R., Hamburger, J. Z., Jiang, K., Kleiner, G., Jurczyszak, D., Matthews, J. C., … Simon, V. (2021). Antibody Responses in Seropositive Persons after a Single Dose of SARS-CoV-2 mRNA Vaccine. *New England Journal of Medicine*, 384(14), 1372–1374. https://doi.org/10.1056/NEJMc2101667

Mahan, V. L. (2014). Clinical Trial Phases. *International Journal of Clinical Medicine*, 05(21), 1374. https://doi.org/10.4236/ijcm.2014.521175

Muralidhara, B. K., Baid, R., Bishop, S. M., Huang, M., Wang, W., & Nema, S. (2016). Critical considerations for developing nucleic acid macromolecule based drug products. *Drug Discovery Today*, 21(3), 430–444. https://doi.org/10.1016/j.drudis.2015.11.012

Palese, P. (1998). RNA virus vectors: Where are we and where do we need to go? *Proceedings of the National Academy of Sciences of the United States of America*, 95(22), 12750–12752.

Pardi, N., Hogan, M. J., Porter, F. W., & Weissman, D. (2018). mRNA vaccines—A new era in vaccinology. *Nature Reviews Drug Discovery*, 17(4), 261–279. https://doi.org/10.1038/nrd.2017.243

Patel, A. K., Kaczmarek, J. C., Bose, S., Kauffman, K. J., Mir, F., Heartlein, M. W., DeRosa, F., Langer, R., & Anderson, D. G. (2019). Inhaled Nanoformulated mRNA Polyplexes for Protein Production in Lung Epithelium. *Advanced Materials*, 31(8), 1805116. https://doi.org/10.1002/adma.201805116

Polack, F. P., Thomas, S. J., Kitchin, N., Absalon, J., Gurtman, A., Lockhart, S., Perez, J. L., Pérez Marc, G., Moreira, E. D., Zerbini, C., Bailey, R., Swanson, K. A., Roychoudhury, S., Koury, K., Li, P., Kalina, W. V., Cooper, D., Frenck, R. W., Hammitt, L. L., ... Gruber, W. C. (2020). Safety and Efficacy of the BNT162b2 mRNA Covid-19 Vaccine. *New England Journal of Medicine*, 383(27), 2603–2615. https://doi.org/10.1056/NEJMoa2034577

Poveda, C., Biter, A. B., Bottazzi, M. E., & Strych, U. (2019). Establishing Preferred Product Characterization for the Evaluation of RNA Vaccine Antigens. *Vaccines*, 7(4), 131. https://doi.org/10.3390/vaccines7040131

Stitz, L., Vogel, A., Schnee, M., Voss, D., Rauch, S., Mutzke, T., Ketterer, T., Kramps, T., & Petsch, B. (2017). *A thermostable messenger RNA based vaccine against rabies*. https://journals.plos.org/plosntds/article?id=10.1371/journal.pntd.0006108&rev=1

Verbeke, R., Lentacker, I., De Smedt, S. C., & Dewitte, H. (2021). The dawn of mRNA vaccines: The COVID-19 case. *Journal of Controlled Release*, 333, 511–520. https://doi.org/10.1016/j.jconrel.2021.03.043

What are protein subunit vaccines and how could they be used against COVID-19? (n.d.). Retrieved May 8, 2021, from https://www.gavi.org/vaccineswork/ what-are-protein-subunit-vaccines-and-how-could-they-be-used-against-covid-19

Yaghchi, C. A., Zhang, Z., Alusi, G., Lemoine, N. R., & Wang, Y. (2015). Vaccinia virus, a promising new therapeutic agent for pancreatic cancer. *Immunotherapy*, 7(12), 1249–1258. https://doi.org/10.2217/imt.15.90

Zeng, C., Zhang, C., Walker, P. G., & Dong, Y. (2020). *Formulation and Delivery Technologies for mRNA Vaccines* (pp. 1–40). Springer. https://doi. org/10.1007/82_2020_217

Zhang, C., Maruggi, G., Shan, H., & Li, J. (2019). Advances in mRNA Vaccines for Infectious Diseases. *Frontiers in Immunology*, 10. https://doi. org/10.3389/fimmu.2019.00594

Chapter 6

Government of Canada. (2021, May 5). Pfizer-BioNTech COVID-19 vaccine: *What you should know.* https://www.canada.ca/en/health-canada/ services/drugs-health-products/covid19-industry/drugs-vaccines-treatments/ vaccines/pfizer-biontech.html

Pfizer. (2020). *A phase 1/2/3, placebo-controlled, randomized, observer-blind, dose-finding study to evaluate the safety, tolerability, immunigenicity, and efficacy of SARS-CoV-2 RNA vaccine candidates against COVID-19 in healthy individuals.* https://cdn.pfizer.com/pfizercom/2020-11/C4591001_Clinical_Protocol_Nov2020.pdf

Pfizer Inc. (2021, February 18). *Pfizer and BioNTech Commence Global Clinical Trial to Evaluate COVID-19 Vaccine in Pregnant Women.* Pfizer. https://www.pfizer.com/news/press-release/press-release-detail/ pfizer-and-biontech-commence-global-clinical-trial-evaluate

Pfizer Inc. (2021, March 31). *Pfizer-BioNTech Announce Positive Topline Results of Pivotal COVID-19 Vaccine Study in Adolescents.* Businesswire. https://www.businesswire.com/news/home/20210331005503/

en/Pfizer-BioNTech-Announce-Positive-Topline-Results-of-Pivot-al-COVID-19-Vaccine-Study-in-Adolescents

Polack, F. P., Thomas, S. J., Kitchin, N., Absalon, J., Gurtman, A., Lock-hart, S., Perez, J. L., Pérez Marc, G., Moreira, E. D., Zerbini, C., Bailey, R., Swanson, K. A., Roychoudhury, S., Koury, K., Li, P., Kalina, W. V., Cooper, D., Frenck, R. W., Hammitt, L. L., ... Gruber, W. C. (2020). Safety and Efficacy of the BNT162b2 mRNA Covid-19 Vaccine. *New England Journal of Medicine*, 383(27), 2603–2615. https://doi.org/10.1056/NEJMoa2034577

U.S. Food and Drug Administration. (2021, April 9). *Pfizer-Bo Tech COVID-19 Vaccine*. https://www.fda.gov/emergency-preparedness-and-response/coronavirus-disease-2019-covid-19/pfizer-biontech-covid-19-vaccine

Walsh, E. E., Frenck, R. W., Falsey, A. R., Kitchin, N., Absalon, J., Gurt-man, A., Lockhart, S., Neuzil, K., Mulligan, M. J., Bailey, R., Swanson, K. A., Li, P., Koury, K., Kalina, W., Cooper, D., Fontes-Garfias, C., Shi, P.-Y., Türeci, Ö., Tompkins, K. R., ... Gruber, W. C. (2020). Safety and Immunogenicity of Two RNA-Based Covid-19 Vaccine Candidates. *New England Journal of Medicine*, 383(25), 2439–2450. https://doi.org/10.1056/NEJMoa2027906

Chapter 7

Canada, S. (2015, October 23). Moderna COVID-19 vaccine: What you should know. Retrieved from aem website: https://www.canada.ca/en/health-canada/services/drugs-health-products/covid19-industry/drugs-vac-cines-treatments/vaccines/moderna.html

CDC. (2020, February 11). COVID-19 and Your Health. Retrieved from Centers for Disease Control and Prevention website: https://www.cdc.gov/coronavirus/2019-ncov/vaccines/different-vaccines/Moderna.html

Clinical Trial Data | Moderna COVID-19 Vaccine (EUA). (n.d.). Retrieved from https://www.modernatx.com/ website: https://www.modernatx.com/covid19vaccine-eua/providers/clinical-trial-data

Moderna Announces Positive Interim Phase 1 Data for its mRNA Vaccine (mRNA-1273) Against Novel

Coronavirus. (2020, May 18). Retrieved from Moderna, Inc. website: https://investors.modernatx.com/news-releases/news-release-details/ moderna-announces-positive-interim-phase-1-data-its-mrna-vaccine

Moderna Announces Publication of Results from the Pivotal Phase 3 Trial of the Moderna COVID-19 Vaccine in The New England Journal of Medicine | Moderna, Inc. (n.d.). Retrieved from investors.modernatx.com website: https:// investors.modernatx.com/news-releases/news-release-details/ moderna-announces-publication-results-pivotal-phase-3-trial

ModernaTX, Inc., & Biomedical Advanced Research and Development Authority. (2021, May 3). A Phase 2a, Randomized, Observer-Blind, Placebo Controlled, Dose-Confirmation Study to Evaluate the Safety, Reactogenicity, and Immunogenicity of mRNA-1273 SARS-COV-2 Vaccine in Adults Aged 18 Years and Older. Retrieved May 17, 2021, from clinicaltrials.gov website: https://clinicaltrials.gov/ct2/show/ NCT04405076?term=NCT04405076&draw=2&rank=1

Partnerships and Researchers: Advancing mRNA - Moderna. (n.d.). Retrieved May 17, 2021, from www.modernatx.com website: https://www. modernatx.com/about-us/mrna-strategic-collaborators

Pipeline | Moderna, Inc. (2018). Retrieved from Modernatx.com website: https://www.modernatx.com/pipeline

Safety and Immunogenicity Study of 2019-nCoV Vaccine (mRNA-1273) for Prophylaxis of SARS-CoV-2 Infection (COVID-19) - Tabular View - ClinicalTrials.gov. (n.d.). Retrieved May 17, 2021, from clinicaltrials.gov website: https://clinicaltrials.gov/ct2/show/record/NCT04283461?view=record

Safety and Immunogenicity Study of 2019-nCoV Vaccine (mRNA-1273) to Prevent SARS-CoV-2 Infection - Full Text View - ClinicalTrials.gov. (n.d.). Retrieved from clinicaltrials.gov website: https://clinicaltrials.gov/ct2/show/ NCT04283461

. (2020). Vaccines and Related Biological Products Advisory Committee Meeting. Retrieved from https://www.fda.gov/media/144434/download

Chapter 8

Amit, S., Regev-Yochay, G., Afek, A., Kreiss, Y., & Leshem, E. (2021). Early rate reductions of SARS-CoV-2 infection and COVID-19 in BNT162b2 vaccine recipients. *The Lancet*, 397(10277), 875–877. https://doi.org/10.1016/S0140-6736(21)00448-7

BBC News. (2021a, April 14). AstraZeneca vaccine: Denmark stops rollout completely. *BBC News*. https://www.bbc.com/news/world-europe-56744474

BBC News. (2021b, April 30). Covid vaccine: Why is the EU suing Astra-Zeneca? *BBC News*. https://www.bbc.com/news/56483766

BBC News. (2021c, May 3). Covax: How will Covid vaccines be shared around the world? *BBC News*. https://www.bbc.com/news/world-55795297

D'Agata, C. (2021, February 27). *One of the strongest weapons against COVID-19 variants may be a vaccine the FDA hasn't approved yet.* CBS News. https://www.cbsnews.com/news/covid-variants-vaccine-oxford-astrazeneca-fda/

Dutta, S. S. (2021, March 10). *What are Adenovirus-Based Vaccines?* News-Medical.Net. https://www.news-medical.net/health/What-are-Adenovirus-Based-Vaccines.aspx

Government of Canada. (2021, April 14). *COVID-19 vaccine extended dose intervals for early vaccine rollout and population protection in Canada: NACI recommendations* [Guidance]. Aem. https://www.canada.ca/en/public-health/services/immunization/national-advisory-committee-on-immuniza-tion-naci/extended-dose-intervals-covid-19-vaccines-early-rollout-popula-tion-protection.html

Irfan, U. (2020, December 30). *The UK approved the Oxford/AstraZeneca Covid-19 vaccine. The US might not get it until April.* Vox. https://www.vox.com/22206498/uk-approves-astrazeneca-vaccine-oxford-covid-19-coronavirus

Kiernan, S., Sethy, P., Shanks, K., & Tohme, S. (2021, March 4). *Vaccine Spheres of Influence Tracker | Think Global Health.* Council on Foreign Relations. https://www.thinkglobalhealth.org/article/vaccine-spheres-influence-tracker

Kupferschmidt, K., & Vogel, G. (2021, May 3). *What's the future of vaccines linked to rare clotting disorders? Science breaks down the latest. Science* I AAAS. https://www.sciencemag.org/news/2021/05/what-s-future-vaccines-linked-rare-clotting-disorders-science-breaks-down-latest

Ministry of Health. (2021a). *Administration of AstraZeneca COVID-19 Vaccine/ COVISHIELD Vaccine.* 13.

Ministry of Health. (2021b). *COVID-19: Vaccine Storage and Handling Guidance.* 37.

Oliver, S. E., Gargano, J. W., Marin, M., Wallace, M., Curran, K. G., Chamberland, M., McClung, N., Campos-Outcalt, D., Morgan, R. L., Mbaeyi, S., Romero, J. R., Talbot, H. K., Lee, G. M., Bell, B. P., & Dooling, K. (2021). The Advisory Committee on Immunization Practices' Interim Recommendation for Use of Moderna COVID-19 Vaccine—United States, December 2020. *MMWR. Morbidity and Mortality Weekly Report*, 69. https://doi.org/10.15585/mmwr.mm695152e1

Østergaard, S. D., Schmidt, M., Horváth-Puhó, E., Thomsen, R. W., & Sørensen, H. T. (2021). Thromboembolism and the Oxford−AstraZeneca COVID-19 vaccine: Side-effect or coincidence? *The Lancet*, 397(10283), 1441−1443. https://doi.org/10.1016/S0140-6736(21)00762-5

Petri, W. (2021, April 4). *How effective is the first shot of the Pfizer or Moderna vaccine?* ASBMB Today. https://www.asbmb.org/asbmb-today/science/040421/how-effective-is-the-first-shot-of-the-pfizer-or-m

Taquet, M., Husain, M., Geddes, J. R., Luciano, S., & Harrison, P. J. (2021). *COVID-19 and cerebral venous thrombosis: A retrospective cohort study of 513,284 confirmed COVID-19 cases.* https://doi.org/10.17605/OSF.IO/H2MT7

Torjesen, I. (2021). Covid-19: Risk of cerebral blood clots from disease is 10 times that from vaccination, study finds. *BMJ*, 373, n1005. https://doi.org/10.1136/bmj.n1005

Voysey, M., Clemens, S. A. C., Madhi, S. A., Weckx, L. Y., Folegatti, P.

M., Aley, P. K., Angus, B., Baillie, V. L., Barnabas, S. L., Bhorat, Q. E., Bibi, S., Briner, C., Cicconi, P., Collins, A. M., Colin-Jones, R., Cutland, C. L., Darton, T. C., Dheda, K., Duncan, C. J. A., ... Zuidewind, P. (2021). Safety and efficacy of the ChAdOx1 nCoV-19 vaccine (AZD1222) against SARS-CoV-2: An interim analysis of four randomised controlled trials in Brazil, South Africa, and the UK. *The Lancet*, 397(10269), 99–111. https://doi.org/10.1016/S0140-6736(20)32661-1

Voysey, M., Clemens, S. A. C., Madhi, S. A., Weckx, L. Y., Folegatti, P. M., Aley, P. K., Angus, B. J., Baillie, V., Barnabas, S. L., Bhorat, Q. E., Bibi, S., Briner, C., Cicconi, P., Clutterbuck, E., Collins, A. M., Cutland, C., Darton, T., Dheda, K., Douglas, A. D., ... Group, O. C. V. T. (2021). *Single dose administration, and the influence of the timing of the booster dose on immunogenicity and efficacy of ChAdOx1 nCoV-19 (AZD1222) vaccine* (SSRN Scholarly Paper ID 3777268). Social Science Research Network. https://doi.org/10.2139/ssrn.3777268

Wise, J. (2021). Covid-19: European countries suspend use of Oxford-AstraZeneca vaccine after reports of blood clots. *BMJ*, 372, n699. https://doi.org/10.1136/bmj.n699

Chapter 9

Balakrishnan, V.S. (2020). The arrival of Sputnik V. *The Lancet Infectious Diseases*, 20, 1128. doi: 10.1016/S1473-3099(20)30709-X

Centers for Disease Control and Prevention. (2021). *Understanding viral vector COVID-19 vaccines*. https://www.cdc.gov/coronavirus/2019-ncov/vaccines/different-vaccines/viralvector.html

European Medicines Agency (n.d.). *What we do*. https://www.ema.europa.eu/en/about-us/what-we-do

Gamaleya Research Institute of Epidemiology and Microbiology. (2020). *An open study of the safety, tolerability and immunogenicity of "Gam-COIVD-Vac Lyo" vaccine against COVID-19*. U.S. National Library of Medicine. https://clinical-trials.gov/ct2/show/NCT04437875?term=Gamaleya&draw=2

Holt, E. (2021). Countries split from EU on COVID-19 vaccines. *The Lancet*,

397, 958. doi: 10.1016/S0140-6736(21)00620-6

Jones, I., & Roy, P. (2021). Sputnik V COVID-19 vaccine candidate appears safe and effective. The Lancet, 397, 642-643. doi: 10.1016/S0140-6736(21)00191-4 Logunov, D. (2021). Safety and efficacy of an rAd26 and rAd5 vector-based heterologous prime-boost COVID-19 vaccine: an interim analysis of a randomised controlled phase 3 trial in Russia. *The Lancet*, 397, 671-681. doi: 10.1016/S0140-6736(21)00234-8

Moore, J.P. (2021). Approaches for optimal use of different COVID-19 vaccines: Issues of viral variants and vaccine efficacy. *The Journal of the American Medical Association*, 325, 1251-1252. doi: 10.1001/jama.2021.3465

Nature. (2021, April 15). Sputnik V vaccine is no match for a fast-spreading variant. https://www-nature-com.ezproxy.library.ubc.ca/articles/d41586-021-00962-8

Oxford University Press. (2021). *Adenovirus*, n. Oxford English Dictionary. https://www-oed-com.ezproxy.library.ubc.ca/view/Entry/2286?redirectedFrom=adenovirus&

Oxford University Press. (2021). *Asthenia*, n. Oxford English Dictionary. https://www-oed-com.ezproxy.library.ubc.ca/view/Entry/12138?redirectedFrom=asthenia#eid

Oxford University Press. (2021). *Polyclinic*, n. Oxford English Dictionary. https://www-oed-com.ezproxy.library.ubc.ca/view/Entry/147107?redirectedFrom=polyclinic#eid

Oxford University Press. (2021). *Telemedicine*, n. Oxford English Dictionary. https://www-oed-com.ezproxy.library.ubc.ca/view/Entry/247413?redirectedFrom=telemedicine#eid

Rogliani, P., Chetta, A., Cazzola, M., & Calzetta, L. (2021). SARS-CoV-2 neutralizing antibodies: A network meta-analysis across vaccines. *Multidisciplinary Digital Publishing Institute*, 9, 227-245. doi: 10.3390/vaccines9030227

Shroff, A. (2020). *What are adenovirus infections?* WebMD. https://www.

webmd.com/children/adenovirus-infections

The Gamaleya Center. (n.d.). *About us*. https://sputnikvaccine.com/about-us/

The Gamaleya Center. (n.d.). *Clinical Trials*. https://sputnikvaccine.com/about-vaccine/clinical-trials/

The Gamaleya Center. (n.d.). *General Information*. https://sputnikvaccine.com/about-vaccine/

World Health Organization (n.d.). *What we do*. https://www.who.int/about/what-we-do

Chapter 10

Blendon, R., Benson, J., & Hero, J. (2014). Public trust in physicians — U.S. medicine in international perspective. *The New England Journal of Medicine*, 371(17), 1570–1572. https://doi.org/10.1056/NEJMp1407373

Cuncic, A. (2020, September 17). *Understanding internal and external validity*. Verywell Mind. https://www.verywellmind.com/internal-and-external-validity-4584479.

Dagan, N., Barda, N., Kepten, E., Miron, O., Perchik, S., Katz, M., Hernán, M., Lipsitch, M., Reis, B., & Balicer, R. (2021). BNT162b2 mRNA Covid-19 vaccine in a nationwide mass vaccination setting. *The New England Journal of Medicine,* 384(15), 1412–1423. https://doi.org/10.1056/NEJMoa2101765

Hewings-Martin , Y., & Cohut, M. (2021, March 15). *COVID-19 vaccines vs. variants: The state of play*. Medical News Today. https://www.medicalnewstoday.com/articles/new-sars-cov-2-variants-how-can-vaccines-be-adapted#-Adapting-vaccines-to-match-variants

Hollingsworth, J. (2021, April 16). *These countries were Covid success stories. Why are they lagging behind on vaccine rollouts?* CNN. https://www.cnn.com/2021/04/15/asia/new-zealand-australia-covid-vaccine-intl-dst-hnk/index.html

Lexchin, J., Mintzes , B., Bero, L., Gagno, M.-A., & Grundy, Q. (2020, October 8). *Canada's COVID-19 Vaccine Task Force needs better transparency about potential conflicts of interest*. The Conversation. https://theconversation. com/canadas-covid-19-vaccine-task-force-needs-better-transparency-about-potential-conflicts-of-interest-147323

MacDonald, N. E., & the SAGE Working Group on Vaccine Hesitancy (2015). Vaccine hesitancy: Definition, scope and determinants. *Vaccine*, 33(34), 4161-4164. https://doi.org/10.1016/j.vaccine.2015.04.036

Mulla, A. M. (2021, April 16). COVID-19: *Kuwait to delay second dose of vaccine amid shortage*. Kuwait. Gulf News. https://gulfnews.com/world/gulf/kuwait/ covid-19-kuwait-to-delay-second-dose-of-vaccine-amid-shortage-1.78936416

Office of the Premier. (2021, January 25). *Ontario adjusts vaccination plan in response to Pfizer-BioNTech shipment delay*s. The Ontario Government. https:// news.ontario.ca/en/release/60091/ontario-adjusts-vaccination-plan-in-re-sponse-to-pfizer-biontech-shipment-delays

Polack, F., Thomas, S., Kitchin, N., Absalon, J., Gurtman, A., Lockhart, S., Perez, J., Pérez Marc, G., Moreira, E., Zerbini, C., Bailey, R., Swanson, K., Roychoudhury, S., Koury, K., Li, P., Kalina, W., Cooper, D., Frenck, R., Hammitt, L., ... Gruber, W. (2020). Safety and efficacy of the BNT162b2 mRNA Covid-19 vaccine. *The New England Journal of Medicine*, 383(27), 2603–2615. https://doi.org/10.1056/NEJMoa2034577

Pope, S. (2021, April 20). *Six people in Vaughan, Ont., injected with saline instead of COVID-19 vaccine*. National Post. https://nationalpost.com/news/ six-people-in-vaughan-ont-injected-with-saline-instead-of-covid-19-vaccine Sallam, M. (2021). COVID-19 vaccine hesitancy worldwide: A concise systematic review of vaccine acceptance rates. *Vaccines (Basel)*, 9(2), 160. https://doi.org/10.3390/vaccines9020160

Schaer, C. (2021, April 16). *Coronavirus: Arab countries struggle with high vaccine hesitancy*. Deutsche Welle. https://www.dw.com/en/ middle-east-covid-vaccine-rollout-hesitancy/a-57227395.

Smith, T. C. (2017, July 18). Vaccine rejection and hesitancy: A review and call to action. *Open Forum Infectious Diseases,* 4(3). https://doi.org/10.1093/ ofid/ofx146

Sweeney, J. F. (2018, April 10). *The eroding trust between patients and physicians*. Medical Economics. https://www.medicaleconomics.com/view/eroding-trust-between-patients-and-physicians.

World Health Organization. (2018). *Ten threats to global health in 2019*. World Health Organization. https://www.who.int/news-room/spotlight/ten-threats-to-global-health-in-2019.

Chapter 11

Rubin, R. (2021, January 26). *Does Vitamin D Deficiency Raise COVID-19 Risk?* JAMA. https://jamanetwork.com/journals/jama/fullarticle/2775003.

AAP FactCheck. (2021, May 7). *False Bill Gates 'depopulate with vaccines' news a conspiracy theory classic - Australian Associated Press*. AustralianAssociatedPress. https://www.aap.com.au/false-bill-gates-depopulate-with-vaccines-news-a-conspiracy-theory-classic/.

Al Jazeera. (2021a, January 4). *Vaccine hesitancy rises in Indonesia amid COVID-19 pandemic*. Coronavirus pandemic News | Al Jazeera. https://www.aljazeera.com/news/2021/1/4/vaccine-hesitancy-rises-in-indonesia-amid-covid-19-pandemic.

Al Jazeera. (2021b, January 22). *UK imams, influencers counter COVID vaccine misinformation*. Coronavirus pandemic News | Al Jazeera. https://www.aljazeera.com/news/2021/1/22/uk-imams-mobilise-to-counter-covid-19-vaccine-disinformation.

Burki T. (2020). The online anti-vaccine movement in the age of COVID-19. *The Lancet. Digital health*, 2(10), e504–e505. https://doi.org/10.1016/S2589-7500(20)30227-2

CCDH. (2021). The Disinformation Dozen. https://252f2edd-1c8b-49f5-9bb2-cb57bb47e4ba.filesusr.com/ugd/f4d9b9_b7cedc0553604720b-7137f8663366ee5.pdf.

Childs, C. E., Calder, P. C., & Miles, E. A. (2019). Diet and Immune Function. Nutrients, 11(8), 1933. https://doi.org/10.3390/nu11081933

Corbie-Smith G, Thomas SB, St. George DMM. Distrust, Race, and Research. *Arch Intern Med.* 2002;162(21):2458–2463. doi:10.1001/archinte.162.21.2458

Dwoskin, E. (2021, February 16). *On social media, vaccine misinformation mixes with extreme faith.* The Washington Post. https://www.washingtonpost.com/technology/2021/02/16/covid-vaccine-misinformation-evangelical-mark-beast/.

FDA. (2021, February 18). *Warning Letter, Mercola.com.* U.S. Food and Drug Administration. https://www.fda.gov/inspections-compliance-enforcement-and-criminal-investigations/warning-letters/mercolacom-llc-607133-02182021.

Funk, C., & Tyson, A. (2021, April 6). *Growing Share of Americans Say They Plan To Get a COVID-19 Vaccine – or Already Have.* Pew Research Center Science & Society. https://www.pewresearch.org/science/2021/03/05/growing-share-of-americans-say-they-plan-to-get-a-covid-19-vaccine--or-already-have/?utm_content=buffer20458&utm_medium=social&utm_source=twitter.com&utm_campaign=buffer.

Goodman, J. G., & Flora, F. (2020, June 26). *Coronavirus: 5G and microchip conspiracies around the world.* BBC News. https://www.bbc.com/news/53191523 .

Heilweil, R. (2020, April 24). *How the 5G coronavirus conspiracy theory went from fringe to mainstream.* Vox. https://www.vox.com/recode/2020/4/24/21231085/coronavirus-5g-conspiracy-theory-covid-facebook-youtube.

Hope, A. (2021, February 14). *Fact-check: Are vaccines halal and kosher?* The Brussels Times. https://www.brusselstimes.com/news/belgium-all-news/154735/fact-check-are-vaccines-halal-and-kosher/.

Rashty, S. (2020, December 31). *More than 70 Jewish doctors say 'no evidence' Covid vaccine causes infertility.* Jewish News. https://jewishnews.timesofisrael.com/jewish-doctors-say-absolutely-no-evidence-covid-19-vaccine-causes-infertility/.

Robeznieks , A. (2020, December 29). *How to overcome COVID-19 vaccine hesitancy among* Black patients. American Medical Association. https://www.ama-assn.org/delivering-care/public-health/ how-overcome-covid-19-vaccine-hesitancy-among-black-patients.

Rodriguez, J. (2021, April 15). *These are the Canadian Muslims dispelling fake news about COVID-19 vaccines.* Coronavirus. https://www.ctvnews.ca/health/ coronavirus/these-are-the-canadian-muslims-dispelling-fake-news-about-covid-19-vaccines-1.5388836.

Satariano, A., & Alba, D. (2020, April 10). *Burning Cell Towers, Out of Baseless Fear They Spread the Virus.* The New York Times. https://www.nytimes. com/2020/04/10/technology/coronavirus-5g-uk.html.

Shirman, Y (2021, March 6) *Black proestants aren't least likely to get a vaccine; white evangelicals are.* Religion News Service. https://religionnews.com/2021/03/05black-protestants-arent-least-likely-to-get-a-vaccine-white-evangelicals-are/.

Smith, A. (2021, January 5). *'5G Covid' mind-control chip diagram is actually a guitar pedal.* The Independent. https://www.independent.co.uk/life-style/ gadgets-and-tech/5g-covid-guitar-pedal-b1782573.html.

Sun, L. H., & Satija, N. (2019, December 23). *A major funder of the anti-vaccine movement has made millions selling natural health products.* The Washington Post. https://www.washingtonpost.com/investigations/2019/10/15/fdc01078-c29c-11e9-b5e4-54aa56d5b7ce_story.html.

Tamayo-Sarver, J. H., Hinze, S. W., Cydulka, R. K., & Baker, D. W. (2003). Racial and ethnic disparities in emergency department analgesic prescription. *American journal of public health*, 93(12), 2067–2073. https://doi. org/10.2105/ajph.93.12.2067

The Children's Hospital of Philadelphia. (2014, November 20). *Vaccine History: Developments by Year.* Children's Hospital of Philadelphia. https:// www.chop.edu/centers-programs/vaccine-education-center/vaccine-history/ developments-by-year.

Ullah, I., Khan, K. S., Tahir, M. J., Ahmed, A., & Harapan, H. (2021, March 11). *Myths and conspiracy theories on vaccines and COVID-19: Potential effect on global vaccine refusals*. Vacunas. https://www.sciencedirect.com/science/article/pii/S1576988721000108.

Williams, J. P. (2021, February 11). *Black Ministers Are Preaching the Gospel About the COVID Vaccine*. U.S. News & World Report. https://www.usnews.com/news/health-news/articles/2021-02-11/black-ministers-preach-the-vaccine-gospel-to-save-their-communities.

Conclusion

Gebre, M. S., Brito, L. A., Tostanoski, L. H., Edwards, D. K., Carfi, A., & Barouch, D. H. (2021). Novel approaches for vaccine development. *Cell*, 184(6), 1589–1603. https://doi.org/10.1016/j.cell.2021.02.030

Jacobson, S. H., Sewell, E. C., & Jokela, J. A. (2007). Survey of vaccine distribution and delivery issues in the USA: from pediatrics to pandemics. *Expert Review of Vaccines*, 6(6), 981–990. https://doi.org/10.1586/14760584.6.6.981

Nikolai, L. A., Meyer, C. G., Kremsner, P. G., & Velavan, T. P. (2020). Asymptomatic SARS Coronavirus 2 infection: Invisible yet invincible. *International Journal of Infectious Diseases*, 100, 112–116. https://doi.org/10.1016/j.ijid.2020.08.076

Verbecke, R., Lentacker, I., De Smedt, S. C., & Dewitte, H. (2021). The dawn of mRNA vaccines: The COVID-19 case. *Journal of Controlled Release*, 333, 511–520. https://doi.org/10.1016/j.jconrel.2021.03.043
World Health Organization. 2020. Clinical Management of COVID-19: Interim Guidance.

www.ingramcontent.com/pod-product-compliance
Lightning Source LLC
Chambersburg PA
CBHW020706270326
41928CB00005B/284